# Practical Teaching in Emergency Medicine

Edited by

Chief Editor
**Robert L. Rogers**

Associate Editors
**Amal Mattu**
**Michael Winters**
**Joseph Martinez**

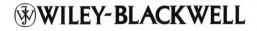

This edition first published 2009, © 2009 by Blackwell Publishing Ltd

Blackwell Publishing was acquired by John Wiley & Sons in February 2007. Blackwell's publishing program has been merged with Wiley's global Scientific, Technical and Medical business to form Wiley-Blackwell.

*Registered office*: John Wiley & Sons Ltd, The Atrium, Southern Gate, Chichester, West Sussex, PO19 8SQ, UK

*Editorial offices*:  9600 Garsington Road, Oxford, OX4 2DQ, UK
The Atrium, Southern Gate, Chichester, West Sussex, PO19 8SQ, UK
111 River Street, Hoboken, NJ 07030-5774, USA

For details of our global editorial offices, for customer services and for information about how to apply for permission to reuse the copyright material in this book please see our website at www.wiley.com/wiley-blackwell

The right of the author to be identified as the author of this work has been asserted in accordance with the Copyright, Designs and Patents Act 1988.

*Library of Congress Cataloging-in-Publication Data*
Practical teaching in emergency medicine / edited by Robert L. Rogers ... [et al.].
    p. ; cm.
    Includes index.
    ISBN 978-1-4051-7622-4
    1. Emergency medicine—Study and teaching. I. Rogers, Robert L.
    [DNLM: 1. Emergency Medicine—education. 2. Emergency Service, Hospital. 3. Teaching—methods. WX 18 P895 2009]
    RC86.7.P687 2009
    616.02'5—dc22
                                                                            2008039506

A catalogue record for this book is available from the British Library.

Set in 9.25/12 pt Meridien by Charon Tec Ltd (A Macmillan Company), Chennai, India (www.macmillansolutions.com)

Printed and bound in Malaysia by KHL Printing Co Sdn Bhd

1  2009

# Dedication

First and foremost, this book is dedicated to my beautiful wife, Tricia, and my two wonderful children, Harrison and Gabriella. Without their love, guidance, and constant support, this book would not have been possible.

I also would like to dedicate the book to all of the educators of emergency medicine in the United States and around the world: may this book inspire others to teach our craft and deliver the very best patient care modern medicine can deliver.

And lastly, to the emergency medicine residents and medical students at The University of Maryland School of Medicine: you are the reason I get up every morning and look forward to working my clinical shifts.

*Rob Rogers*

My thanks to my family for their constant support; my colleagues, residents, and students for their inspiration to teach and to learn; and to all those who spend their time teaching emergency medicine around the world ... may your efforts continue to help our specialty flourish.

*Amal Mattu*

To the medical students and emergency medicine residents at the University of Maryland for making me look forward to my shifts, and to Lisa, Nicholas, Dylan, and Luke for making me happy to go home.

*Joseph Martinez*

To my wonderful wife Erika and our beautiful children Hayden and Emma, thank you. None of my accomplishments would have been possible without your enduring love and endless support. The three of you are my source of inspiration. To the residents and faculty at the University of Maryland, you are an amazing group of educators and it is my privilege to be your colleague.

*Michael Winters*

# Contents

Editors and Contributors, ix
Preface, xv

**Section 1 Background/Introduction**

**Chapter 1** Adult learners in the emergency department, 3
*Ellen J. O'Connell, Kurt C. Kleinschmidt*

**Chapter 2** Obstacles to teaching in the emergency department, 16
*Esther K. Choo, Jeffrey A. Tabas*

**Chapter 3** Teaching and patient care in emergency medicine, 24
*Michael A. Bohrn, David A. Kramer*

**Section 2 Teaching in the Emergency Department**

**Chapter 4** Bedside teaching in the emergency department, 35
*Kevin G. Rodgers*

**Chapter 5** Teaching procedures: beyond "see one, do one, teach one", 48
*Mercedes Torres, Siamak Moayedi*

**Chapter 6** Providing feedback in the emergency department, 60
*David A. Wald, Esther K. Choo*

**Chapter 7** The computer as a teaching tool, 72
*Joshua S. Broder*

**Chapter 8** Teaching the intangibles: professionalism and interpersonal skills/communication, 87
*David K. Zich, James G. Adams*

**Section 3 Teaching Specific Groups**

**Chapter 9** Teaching medical students, 105
*David E. Manthey*

**Chapter 10** Teaching trainees from other services in the emergency department, 114
*Michelle Lin*

**Chapter 11** The education of resident physicians in emergency medicine: A United States perspective, 125
*Stuart P. Swadron, William K. Mallon*

**Chapter 12** Teaching physicians in training how to teach, 146
*Carey D. Chisholm*

**Section 4 Improving as an Educator in Emergency Medicine**

**Chapter 13** Characteristics of great teachers, 159
*Jennifer Avegno, Peter DeBlieux*

**Chapter 14** Effective presentation skills, 168
*Joseph R. Lex Jr.*

**Chapter 15** Small group discussion skills, 180
*Matthew D. Deibel, Mary Jo Wagner*

**Chapter 16** Faculty development as a guide for becoming a better teacher, 192
*Gloria J. Kuhn*

**Section 5 Teaching Techniques and Strategies**

**Chapter 17** Strategies for effective clinical emergency department teaching, 213
*Glen Bandiera, Shirley Lee*

**Chapter 18** Pearls and pitfalls in teaching: what works, what doesn't?, 225
*Brian Clyne, David G. Lindquist*

Index, 235

# Editors and Contributors

## Chief Editor

**Robert L. Rogers**
Assistant Professor of Emergency Medicine and Medicine
Director of Undergraduate Medical Education
Department of Emergency Medicine
The University of Maryland School of Medicine
Baltimore, MD, USA

## Associate Editors

**Amal Mattu**
Associate Professor of Emergency Medicine
Director, Emergency Medicine Residency
Director, Faculty Development Fellowship
Department of Emergency Medicine
The University of Maryland School of Medicine
Baltimore, MD, USA

**Michael Winters**
Assistant Professor of Emergency Medicine and Medicine
Director, Critical Care Education
Co-Director, Emergency Medicine/Internal Medicine
Critical Care Residency Program
Department of Emergency Medicine
The University of Maryland School of Medicine
Baltimore, MD, USA

**Joseph Martinez**
Assistant Professor of Emergency Medicine and Medicine
Assistant Dean for Student Affairs
Department of Emergency Medicine
The University of Maryland School of Medicine
Baltimore, MD, USA

## Contributors

**James G. Adams**
Professor and Chair
Department of Emergency Medicine
Northwestern University
Feinberg School of Medicine
Northwestern Memorial Hospital
Chicago, IL, USA

**Jennifer Avegno**
Medical Student Clerkship Director
LSUHSC Section of Emergency Medicine
New Orleans, LA, USA

**Glen Bandiera**
Assistant Professor, Clinician Educator, FRCP(EM) Residency
  Director
Department of Medicine
University of Toronto, *and*
Staff Emergency Physician, Trauma Team Leader, Director of
  Postgraduate Medical Education
St. Michael's Hospital
Toronto, Ontario, Canada

**Michael A. Bohrn**
Associate Residency Program Director, Clinical Assistant
  Professor
Department of Emergency Medicine
York Hospital
York, PA, USA

**Joshua S. Broder**
Duke University Division of Emergency Medicine
Duke University Medical Center
Durham, NC, USA

**Carey D. Chisholm**
Professor of Emergency Medicine, Emergency Medicine
  Residency Director
Indiana University School of Medicine
Indianapolis, Indiana, USA

**Esther K. Choo**
Research Fellow & Clinical Instructor
Department of Emergency Medicine
Oregon Health & Science University
Portland, OR, USA

**Brian Clyne**
Assistant Professor of Emergency Medicine
Director, Residency Program
Department of Emergency Medicine
The Warren Alpert Medical School of Brown University
Providence, RI, USA

**Peter M.C. DeBlieux**
Director of Resident and Faculty Development
Section of Emergency Medicine, Professor of Clinical Medicine
Staff Physician, Pulmonary/Critical Care
New Orleans, LA, USA

**Matthew D. Deibel**
Emergency Physician,
Emergency Care Center,
Covenant HealthCare
Saginaw, *and*
Assistant Clinical Professor
Program in Emergency Medicine
Michigan State University College of Human Medicine
East Lansing, MI, USA

**Kurt C. Kleinschmidt**
Associate Professor, Associate Medical Director, Toxicology
  Fellowship Director
Division of Emergency Medicine
University of Texas Southwestern Medical Center
Parkland Health & Hospital System
Dallas, TX, USA

**David A. Kramer**
Program Director and Vice Chair, Clinical Associate Professor
Department of Emergency Medicine
York Hospital
York, PA, USA

**Gloria J. Kuhn**
Vice Chair Academic Affairs
Department of Emergency Medicine
Wayne State University
Detroit, MI, USA

**Shirley Lee**
Assistant Professor
Department of Family and Community Medicine
University of Toronto, *and*
Assistant Director – Education, Schwartz-Reisman
  Emergency Centre
Mt. Sinai Hospital
Toronto, Ontario, Canada

**Joseph R. Lex Jr.**
Assistant Professor of Emergency Medicine
Temple University School of Medicine
Philadelphia, PA, USA

**Michelle Lin**
Associate Program Director
UCSF-SFGH Emergency Medicine Residency Program
Assistant Clinical Professor of Medicine
University of California San Francisco
San Francisco General Hospital, Emergency Services
San Francisco, CA, USA

**David G. Lindquist**
Assistant Professor of Emergency Medicine
Department of Emergency Medicine
The Warren Alpert Medical School of Brown University
Providence, RI, USA

**William K. Mallon**
Director of International Emergency Medicine
Associate Professor
Department of Emergency Medicine
Los Angeles County/USC Medical Center
Keck School of Medicine of the University of
  Southern California
Los Angeles, CA, USA

**David E. Manthey**
Department of Emergency Medicine
Associate Professor of Emergency Medicine
Wake Forest University School of Medicine
Medical Center Boulevard
Winston-Salem, NC, USA

**Siamak Moayedi**
Assistant Professor
Department of Emergency Medicine
University of Maryland, School of Medicine
Baltimore, MD, USA

**Ellen J. O'Connell**
Assistant Professor
Division of Emergency Medicine
University of Texas Southwestern Medical Center
Parkland Health & Hospital System
Dallas, TX, USA

**Kevin G. Rodgers**
Professor of Clinical Emergency Medicine
Co-Program Director
Emergency Medicine Residency
Indiana University School of Medicine
Indianapolis, IN, USA

**Stuart P. Swadron**
Vice-Chair of Education and Program Director
Department of Emergency Medicine
Associate Professor, Keck School of Medicine of the
  University of Southern California
Los Angeles County/USC Medical Center
Los Angeles, CA, USA

**Jeffrey A. Tabas**
Director Performance Improvement
San Francisco General Hospital Emergency Services
Associate Professor, UCSF School of Medicine
San Francisco, CA, USA

**Mercedes Torres**
Assistant Professor
University of Maryland, School of Medicine
Baltimore, MD, USA

**Mary Jo Wagner**
Program Director, Synergy Medical Education Alliance/Michigan
  State University
Emergency Medicine Residency Program
Saginaw, MI, USA
Associate Professor, Program in Emergency Medicine
Michigan State University College of Human Medicine
East Lansing, MI, USA

**David A. Wald**
Director of Undergraduate Medical Education
Associate Professor of Emergency Medicine
Department of Emergency Medicine
Temple University School of Medicine
Wynnewood, PA, USA

**David K. Zich**
Assistant Professor of Medicine
Departments of Emergency Medicine and Internal Medicine
Northwestern University
Feinberg School of Medicine
Northwestern Memorial Hospital
Chicago, IL, USA

# Preface

The emergency department (ED) is one of the most interesting and rewarding teaching venues in the house of medicine. No other environment offers such a rich blend of undifferentiated patient presentations and diseases. However, because of this diversity, the ED is also one of the most difficult places to teach. Many of our patients are desperately ill, and we must often reset our priorities quickly to meet their clinical demands. In this environment, emergency medicine educators are challenged to provide quality education for medical students and physicians-in-training.

Emergency medicine attendings who wish to hone their teaching skills can find a number of textbooks on educational strategies written by physicians from other disciplines. However, until now, they have not had access to a text written by emergency medicine physicians on methods of teaching that are directly applicable to our specialty. This book was compiled to meet that need. Its purpose is to provide educators in emergency medicine with a resource on best practices in teaching the art of emergency medicine. The contents are organized around the topics of teaching specific groups of learners, teaching in the emergency department, improving as an educator in emergency medicine, and appreciating various teaching techniques and strategies.

The chapter contributors are widely regarded as leaders in the field of emergency medicine education and faculty development. Authors were given free rein to develop their chapters and write in their own style. They were asked to present their personal views on how to successfully teach the art of emergency medicine, rather than review evidence-based guidelines regarding medical education. As a result, most of the chapters have few references. This first-person approach to a multi-authored textbook yields a compilation that varies in style from chapter to chapter and exposes the reader to a variety of communication techniques. The editors hope that readers find useful models within these pages as they refine their own methods for teaching in the spectrum of venues where emergency medicine is taught.

Inherent to the teaching and the practice of emergency medicine are specific challenges not found in other specialties – the unknowns of the ED, the need to identify life- and limb-threatening conditions, the pressure to solve problems and find solutions quickly, the orchestration of clinical specialists and ancillary services. Because of these unique demands of our practice, books written by clinicians from other disciplines may be helpful but not complete for us. *Practical Teaching in Emergency Medicine* was written by emergency medicine physicians for emergency medicine physicians. We hope you find it to be a valuable resource toward teaching the art of practicing our beloved specialty.

Robert L. Rogers, M.D.
Chief Editor
Practical Teaching in Emergency Medicine

# SECTION 1
# Background/Introduction

# CHAPTER 1

# Adult learners in the emergency department

*Ellen J. O'Connell, Kurt C. Kleinschmidt*
Division of Emergency Medicine, University of Texas Southwestern Medical Center,
Parkland Health & Hospital System, Dallas, TX, USA

## Introduction

"Why do I have to learn this?" is a common complaint among school-aged students while learning dreaded subjects. The teacher's answer is usually, "Because I said so." The standard student retort to this is, "Well, I'll never have to use this in the real world."

Adulthood has arrived; the real world. Unlike our youthful days when educational subjects were forced upon us, most adults seek to learn because of a motivation to do so. Adults seek experiences that have an identifiable impact on life. However, the motivation for adult learning is not always from within; external forces also affect motivation. Adults sometimes seek education, not because they are excited about the subject, but because they know it is in their best interest. Adults also seek learning so as to better deal with the real world. This is the basic difference of perspective toward learning between an adult and a child.

The purpose of this chapter is to explore the principles of adult education as it applies to teaching in the emergency department (ED). Examples of these principles will be applied to this specific clinical setting. The terms "learner" and "physician-in-training" refer to anyone in the position of learning. The "teacher," "instructor," or "educator" is the person at any level of training who is in the teaching role.

*Practical Teaching in Emergency Medicine*, 1st edition. Edited by R Rogers, A Mattu, M Winters & J Martinez. ©2009 Blackwell Publishing, ISBN: 9781405176224

## Learning theories

Physiologically, learning is building and strengthening the synapses in the brain. The details are complex and unknown. This unknown territory has resulted in the development of many learning theories, including three recognized classic theories [1]. Each of these theories creates an impact on curriculum design, teaching, and evaluation. Most educators use elements from each theory in any given situation rather than strictly adhering to one particular style.

Behaviorism is the learning theory commonly associated with the Pavlovian response: a subject performs a behavior, receives a positive result, and the behavior is reinforced. If the result is negative, then the behavior is discouraged and eventually eliminated. The behaviorist does not focus on the thought processes of the learner, but only on the response to a stimulus.

The cognitive learning theory is the opposite of behaviorism. It focuses on the learner's thought processes instead of a response to a stimulus. The interest is in how the learner integrates new information and applies it to new situations.

The third classic learning theory is constructivism. In this theory, the learner builds (or constructs) new ideas based on existing knowledge. Constructivism also focuses on how students interact and learn from each other, as well as from their educators.

## Learning as a child

*Pedagogy* refers to the learning style of children. Its literal translation from Greek is "to lead the child." This is a teacher-centered style of learning. Because children are not thought to have sufficient experience to know what they need to learn, their educators make these decisions for them. Instructors decide what material to teach and how to teach it. Young students have little choice as to the content of their curriculum. Decisions and information flow 100% from instructor to student.

Aspects of the pedagogical style also apply to some adult learning situations. For example, during the preclinical years of medical school, adult students also have no choice regarding the content of their curriculum. However, unlike secondary school students, adults have chosen to do this curriculum because of their motivation to become physicians. The curriculum is a means to an identifiable end, providing motivation.

## Learning as an adult

As the study of learning advanced, adult learning enthusiasts recognized that children and adults receive and process new information differently. This recognition suggested that adults should be taught differently, prompting radical changes in adult education in many institutions. In the mid-1950s, Malcolm Knowles began publishing his work on adult education, which at the time was an underexplored subject. He popularized the term *andragogy*, which he defined as "the art and science of helping adults learn." He observed that adults needed to be involved in their education rather than being "led" to it. While childhood learning is teacher centered, adult learning is student centered.

Much of the adult learning theory stems from five assumptions about adult learners developed by Knowles (Table 1.1). The assumptions reflect that adults are self-directed learners who seek information independently. They reconcile new information with their existing knowledge base, and they seek to apply it immediately to a known problem. It is important to note that these assumptions have not yet been validated.

Pedagogical learning is based upon discrete subjects, such as math, history, and spelling; or anatomy, cell biology, and pharmacology. This is appropriate for building lower levels of cognition, and for the development of a foundation of knowledge. However, applying very basic knowledge, acquired in a pedagogical style, to real-world problems is more difficult. Adult learning is more problem centered, an approach in which the learner pulls multiple bits of basic information from multiple, discrete subjects to solve a problem.

Problem-centered learning is very relevant in the ED. For example, the ED physician, faced with a female who has right lower quadrant abdominal pain, simultaneously gives attention

**Table 1.1** Malcolm Knowles' adult learning assumptions.

| |
|---|
| Adults are self-directed and autonomous |
| Adults have life experiences that need to be respected |
| Adults desire to learn tasks related to everyday life |
| Adults are problem centered and seek to immediately apply learned material |
| Adults are motivated by internal drives rather than external factors |

Refs [6, 8].

to all systems that may cause pain in this region, thus deciding: "Is this gastrointestinal (appendicitis, gastroenteritis), gynecologic (ectopic pregnancy, ovarian torsion, pelvic inflammatory disease), genitourinary (ureterolithiasis, pyelonephritis), vascular (aortic dissection), or other (shingles)?" The physician combines basic knowledge of these different systems and conditions with clinical experience to narrow the diagnostic possibilities and begin the appropriate evaluation.

Before embracing Knowles' theories blindly, one must note that there are many criticisms of Knowles' work. The lack of data used to formulate the assumptions is commonly cited [2–5]. This is particularly concerning in medicine's current culture of evidence-based practice. Additionally, Knowles' work is often considered "theory." This is an inappropriate use of this word, since a scientific theory is one that has been rigorously tested, and these learning assumptions have not.

Norman [2] questions at what point a student optimally transitions from a child to an adult learning style. It is not likely an age-based phenomenon, as chronological and mental ages are not always congruent. He suggests that the time of the transition is not effected by an internal condition of the learner, but rather by the change in learning style needed to meet a new pressure or situation.

Some have suggested that the motivation for adult learning is rarely exclusively internal; that motivation often stems from external forces [3, 5]. Adults may only acknowledge their conscious internal motivation, neglecting a subconscious external motivation. For example, physicians must receive continuing medical education (CME) in order to maintain their certification. A physician may satisfy an internal drive to learn more about dental emergencies by attending a lecture on this topic at a conference; the external motivation of receiving CME credits is also satisfied by attending this lecture.

The assumption that adult learning is all self-directed is also debatable [2, 5]. Self-direction is a quality of a mature learner. A young learner may possess this quality, whereas a chronologically older student may not. In addition, before indulging into any self-directed learning, students must do self-assessments to identify their weaknesses. However, young students often perform inadequate self-assessment. The drive to learn is partly fed by success. Consequently, students are more likely to study topics with which they are familiar, feeding the hunger for success rather than focusing on weak areas. Adult learners facing new subjects may need a little "pedagogical guidance" from instructors.

Another criticism of Knowles' work is that he did not comment on the use of reflection in learning [5]. In reflection, the learner considers the new material, integrating the new material with preexisting knowledge and resolving conflicts between new and old information. The learner can also consider how to approach a task the next time, based on successes and mistakes in the first experience. Taking time to reflect upon a newly learned topic serves to ingrain the material into one's mind, strengthening the newly formed synapses.

## Educating adults

Adults are experienced learners who derive part of their identity from life experiences. Adult learning is enhanced when educators demonstrate *respect* to the adults, as well as to their experiences. Any dismissal of the learner's experience is perceived as a rejection of himself or herself [6]. With the learners' cadre of life experiences come well-established, difficult-to-break habits [6]. Despite their motivation to learn, adults are generally resistant toward changing their habits. Educators must balance respect for the learners' experiences with needed modifications of problem habits. Failure to balance this may risk alienating the learners.

Dependence on the teacher within a pedagogical structure is counterintuitive to adult learners. Adult learners seek to solve problems on their own using previous experience. Instructors of adult students are seen as facilitators, not teachers. Facilitators are guides who do not merely hand out information but who help students to develop their own questions and to find their own answers. This develops student self-reliance and skills that will be useful in solving future problems. Knowles and others have developed recommendations for these facilitators of adult students [7, 8], detailed with examples in the following section.

## Adult learning in the ED

The ED is a very rich, problem-based, learning environment. Most emergency medicine (EM) physicians are "action oriented" people who say, "I learn best by doing," or "I learn on my feet." The ED provides the ideal setting for such learning. Patients are present here with a complaint to be diagnosed, not a diagnosis to be managed. The educational moments are "live;" they are "now." Skilled educators exploit these attributes of the ED, incorporating principles of adult education to create rich learning experiences for the young physicians.

However, the ED is not a "comfortable" learning environment. Constant distractions are normal. Another significant barrier to education in the ED is time. Faculties are clearly under increasing pressures to see more patients, further limiting the time for teaching. The balancing of time between patient care and teaching is just another ED triage; only that this is "time triage." Not all cases need to be an educational moment, nor must every aspect of each case be dissected to provide thorough teaching. Educators must choose their moments.

**Set the environment**

There are two environments to optimize for learning: physical and interpersonal. The physical environment of the ED is a constant assault on all the senses, resulting in an array of distractions that is unparalleled in the world of education. Patients are constantly coming and going whereas providers are ever darting about. Noise emanates from patients, monitors, radios, telephones, overhead speakers, and chatter between coworkers. The lighting is harsh. The department is never big enough, with patients overflowing from rooms into hallway beds or large rooms with chairs. Nurses and physicians also have to battle for computer space; if there are enough computers, there is not enough counter space. Supplies run short, textbooks are old, and "who took the last cup of coffee without making a new pot?" interruptions are frequent. New learners in the ED also face shear intimidation. Despite these inordinate challenges, learners must focus on good quality, one-at-a-time, patient care. It would seem impossible to also get the learner to focus on educational moments, one-at-a-time. Teachers in the ED must choose their moments among the distractions. It is important to "read" your learner to see if they are ready for educational moments. If a student is too distracted with a current situation, you cannot effectively teach. Save the pearl for later.

The interpersonal or relationship setting is the most important piece in the entire educational endeavor. As noted earlier, adults have years of experience for which they expect and deserve respect. Establishing an open and respectful relationship with the adult learner is the most important initial step in providing adult education. It is this relationship that encourages learners to come to their teachers, and also makes the teachers approachable. Simply, learning will not occur if the students do not want to approach or hear from the teacher. Since in the teaching ED, physicians-in-training have to present their cases, it seems that the learners have no choice but to come to the teachers. However, if the learners do not have a good relationship with the teacher, they will modify their presentations in ways to minimize exposure to the instructors. When faculties try to teach in the setting of poor relationships, learners will be minimally receptive. Tension easily worsens with each encounter. Various reviews have been done that describe the characteristics of

**Table 1.2** Characteristics of effective teachers.

---

*Enthusiasm*
Psychosocial focus
- Stresses relationships with patients and staff
- Patient centered
- Understands personal perspectives and social values
- Humanitarian

*Identifies self as a teacher*
Communication skills
- Listens to students
- Rapport with students
- Nonthreatening (approachable)
- Questions carefully done
- Clear and lucid
- Organized

Role model actions
- Positive
- Responds to teaching needs
- Listens to patients
- Rapport with patients
- Emphasizes relationships
- Emphasizes psychosocial aspects of cases
- Knowledgeable
- Clinically competent

Encourages education and independence
- Actively involves students
- Provides direction and feedback
- Stimulates intellectual curiosity
- Promotes self-direction

---

Refs [10–15].

good teaching faculty (Table 1.2). Upon review of these characteristics, it can be noted that they are all based upon the establishment of an open and respectful relationship with the learners.

## Set goals

Goals are the centerpiece of education. Adult learners should assist in determining their learning goals as much as possible. Learners can reflect on their existing knowledge and identify gaps that must be filled. This strengthens their internal motivation and develops a sense of responsibility for their education. In an ED, goals can be established any time including orientation, the beginning of a shift, or on the fly as a resuscitation is about to begin. However, learners cannot determine these goals alone. Goals may result after negotiation between the student and the teacher. Educator input is also valuable in ensuring that learners have set specific, achievable, and measurable goals.

During orientation, ask off-service rotators and medical students to consider what they hope to achieve during their time in the ED. Many will have very limited goals. Challenge them to expand their thinking, since the ED is a place for non-EM physicians to face problems outside their chosen practice. Consider having the physicians-in-training establish a goal for the day at the beginning of a shift. This may be a part of the history, such as asking each patient the nature of his or her employment. Alternatively, the learner can enhance physical exam skills, such as carefully listening to cardiac murmurs in each patient. Educators can help the learners recognize unrealistic goals, such as improving chest tube placement.

Some non-EM rotators may desire to learn everything related to EM while in the ED. However, non-EM physicians-in-training often present unique challenges because they may have goals for the rotation that are different than the teacher's desire to teach them "emergency medicine." An orthopedics physician-in-training may only seek musculoskeletal injuries, whereas an internal medicine physician-in-training may target lengthy, inpatient work-ups on ED patients at a rate of one patient per hour. It may be impossible to "make" these physicians-in-training meet the instructors' desired goals. Thus, negotiation becomes an important part of the process. Attempts to force certain goals upon some learners will only result in frustration for all. Admittedly, not all would agree with this, as some feel all rotators should be taught everything related to EM.

Learners may struggle to choose goals. Instructors can assist by asking questions to identify areas of weakness. For example, a physician-in-training may say, "I hate eye complaints." Questioning reveals that this aversion is due to a lack of comfort with performing a complete eye exam. If the physician-in-training is in EM, the instructor can ensure this is taught during the shift. If the learner in non-EM has no interest in learning the details of the eye exam, then time might be wasted in trying to do so. It might be the appropriate time to probe again and find a weakness that is of interest.

**Plan and implement new material**
Involving learners in planning educational activities has many benefits, including assisting the facilitators in identifying possible problems before they become definite issues. Facilitators can redirect learners when they are off-track and provide recommendations for problem solving resources.

This technique applies easily to procedures. All providers have preferred approaches for different procedures. Physicians-in-training may not have broad enough exposure to different techniques. Asking one to try a different technique or approach may result in some resistance. Querying, "Why do you think it may be valuable to know how to place internal jugular central lines rather than just femoral lines?" may help the learner realize that not all approaches are available in all patients. Consequently the physician-in-training gains motivation for learning a new approach as well. Having learners discuss about procedures before they are done reinforces the appropriate steps and identifies knowledge gaps before undertaking the tasks. Being present during the procedure is ideal though often impractical. It is reasonable to consider that different procedures have different levels of risks and thus different levels of need for physical presence by the teacher.

Implementing education is difficult during the middle of a procedure or resuscitation. Educators naturally want to intervene and/or make comments; but doing so may be at the expense of the physician-in-training. These moments require the difficult balance of patient care with education. Intervention by the teacher can embarrass the learner, potentially harming the student–teacher relationship. However, patient care is a very important consideration. There is no easy answer for these potentially conflicting interests. The best consideration is that there are no absolutes; neither should always be the dominant one. Minor mistakes by a physician-in-training can be just as acceptable as the teacher stepping in at a truly life threatening moment. For those who practice EM, we recognize that the truly life threatening moments, where key decisions in a matter of very few minutes will truly affect life, are few. Usually, there is time for the teacher to discuss the situation with the learner, facilitating and guiding. An excellent location for the teacher is right behind the learner. This location enables the teacher to quietly make comments to the learner, enabling him or her to remain "in-charge." Once the life threatening moment has passed, then even the minor mistakes can be addressed during the postresuscitation review.

Another implementation opportunity occurs when a topic is raised to which the educator has a canned, brief presentation. Many teachers have a variety of topics, such as causes and evaluation of syncope, management of asthma when standard medications fail, emergency causes of chest pain, or how to interpret a chest X-ray. Educators keep these discussions fine-tuned and ready for use when the appropriate moments occur. These lectures are brief, usually no longer than 3 minutes. This aids the learner in retaining the information (by avoiding information overload), as well as avoids significant delay patient care.

### Evaluate

By evaluating their learning experiences, adult learners identify ongoing knowledge gaps and recognize whether goals were met. These evaluations do not use formalized exams; rather may be done with a brief discussion between the learner and the teacher. Reviewing key aspects of patient encounters can be very helpful, especially if it includes comments on previously established goals.

The verbal discussion (or evaluation) is routine during standard patient presentations by physicians-in-training. After the presentation of a history and physical condition, ask a physician-in-training to formulate a differential diagnosis, what he or she wants to do from this point, and the thought processes behind both. This gives the educator insight into the learner's understanding of the patient's illness, as well as whether the learner has an appropriate diagnostic approach or not. This also is a chance for the educator to guide the learner back on track should the plan not seem appropriate based on the presentation.

A similar recap should take place after the physician-in-training has undertaken a specific challenge, such as a new approach in a procedure. A similar query of, "How did you think this went, what did you learn, what would you have done differently?" gives the learner a moment to evaluate his or her own performance, again reinforcing the new material.

## Role model

> Example is not the main thing in influencing others. It is the only thing.
>
>                                                    Albert Schweitzer

Role modeling is very important to education in the ED. In some ways, this is the easiest education that teachers deliver. It requires little thought or planning, and mostly the teachers being the role model themselves. Amazingly, EM teachers may be unaware that they are role modeling. Physicians in any senior position should be aware of their behavior being emulated at any time [9]. Thus, in other words, this can be the most difficult part of being a teacher, as you are onstage 100% of the time. An EM teacher's every action or word is interpreted, and the interpretation may be very different than what was intended by the teacher. Every verbal interaction is seen by at least one person, and the patterns soon become clear. The disgusted look given to the technician for delivering the latest electrocardiogram is generally witnessed. The challenge is to be the best human we can be as much of the time as possible. It is no surprise that most positive human attributes are the same as the characteristics of an effective teacher discussed earlier (Table 1.2).

Observation of a teacher's history and the physical exam of a patient can be illuminating to a learner. The clinician's techniques can be incorporated into their own routines: subtle uses of humor, good eye contact, or the shake of a hand. Educators can then point out findings to the learner and explain why certain questions were used.

One of the most important items that can be role modeled is how the teacher thinks. For example, after having heard the differential diagnosis and plan from the physician-in-training, the teacher explains his or her differential and plan loudly. This is more than just stating a differential and plan. It is very powerful for the learner to see the educator model his or her thought processes by "thinking out loud."

An instructor may also model an experience, which is difficult to teach, such as conveying to the family the death of a loved one. The educator can identify ahead of time specific techniques, such as bringing a chaplain or nurse as an escort and clearly stating that the loved one died. This serves as cues for which the learner should be watching as the role model proceeds in his or her task. Afterward, the instructor can ask the learner for his or her thoughts on the experience. This serves both as feedback for the instructor and to embed the experience in the learner's mind.

## Conclusion

To summarize, adult learners are self-directed and goal oriented, seeking information that they can readily apply. The ED provides many appropriate educational moments for adult learners. Educators can seize these moments by helping the learner set goals, serve as a guide on the learner's path to learning but not spoon-feed answers, and help the learner evaluate his or her performance to further solidify the new information.

---

### Summary points

- Adult learners have internal motivation, frequently combined with external motivation, to actively seek new information, reconcile new information with existing knowledge, and plan to rapidly apply information to a problem.
- Reflection on newly learned material or tasks serves to integrate the new material into a learner's brain, making it more readily retrievable in future experiences.
- Adult learners need from their educators respect for their existing knowledge base.
- Setting a positive interpersonal environment will help overcome the ED's physical impediments to learning.
- Physicians-in-training must develop learning goals; learners must evaluate both independently and with their educator how those goals have been met.
- Educators must be open to identify opportunities for learning in the ED, such as patient presentations by physicians-in-training, procedures, and resuscitations.
- Educators should realize they are always role models; their behavior, both positive and negative, is always on display for absorption by learners.

# References

1. Williamson KB, Gunderman RB, Cohen MD, *et al.* Learning theory in radiology education. *Radiology* 2004; 233(1): 15–18.
2. Norman GR. The adult learner: a mythical species. *Acad Med* 1999; 74(8): 886–889.
3. Misch DA. Andragogy and medical education: are medical students internally motivated to learn? *Adv Health Sci Educ Theory Pract* 2002; 7(2): 153–160.
4. Ende J. Learning about learning. *J Gen Intern Med* 1995; 10(3): 172–173.
5. Mann KV. The role of educational theory in continuing medical education: has it helped us? *J Contin Educ Health Prof* 2004; 24(Suppl 1): S22–S30.
6. David TJ, Patel L. Adult learning theory, problem based learning, and paediatrics. *Arch Dis Child* 1995; 73(4): 357–363.
7. Curry RH, Hershman WY, Saizow RB. Learner-centered strategies in clerkship education. *Am J Med* 1996; 100(6): 589–595.
8. Kaufman DM. Applying educational theory in practice. *BMJ* 2003; 326(7382): 213–216.
9. Maudsley RF. Role models and the learning environment: essential elements in effective medical education. *Acad Med* 2001; 76(5): 432–434.
10. Hilliard RI. The good and effective teacher as perceived by pediatric residents and by faculty. *Am J Dis Child* 1990; 144(10): 1106–1110.
11. Irby D, Rakestraw P. Evaluating clinical teaching in medicine. *J Med Educ* 1981; 56(3): 181–186.
12. Molodysky E, Sekelja N, Lee C. Identifying and training effective clinical teachers – new directions in clinical teacher training. *Aust Fam Physician* 2006; 35(1–2): 53–55.
13. Schor EL, Grayson M. Outstanding clinical teachers: methods, characteristics and behaviors. *Res Med Educ* 1984; 23: 271–276.
14. Wright SM, Kern DE, Kolodner K, *et al.* Attributes of excellent attending-physician role models. *N Engl J Med* 1998; 339(27): 1986–1993.
15. Mattern WD, Weinholtz D, Friedman CP. The attending physician as teacher. *N Engl J Med* 1983; 308(19): 1129–1132.

# CHAPTER 2

# Obstacles to teaching in the emergency department

*Esther K. Choo[1], Jeffrey A. Tabas[2]*
[1]*Research Fellow & Clinical Instructor, Department of Emergency Medicine, Oregon Health & Science University, Portland, OR, USA*
[2]*Associate Professor of Emergency Medicine, UCSF School of Medicine Attending Physician, San Francisco General Hospital Emergency Services, San Francisco, CA, USA*

The emergency department (ED) offers what may be the greatest educational opportunity in medicine. Patients present with undifferentiated conditions from every field of medicine, requiring sophistication in history taking and physical examination, laboratory and radiologic testing, multitasking and prioritization, as well as interpersonal interactions. However, the ED also throws significant obstacles in the way of instructors who attempt to utilize this potential treasure trove of education. Many of these obstacles are inherent to the ED – such as chronic time limitations, frequent interruptions, and lack of physical space for teaching – while others are common to instructors across medical specialties and only exacerbated by the ED environment.

## Obstacles inherent to the ED

Educators in the ED often cite lack of time as the major obstacle to their teaching during a shift. While balancing patient care and teaching is always a challenge, nowhere is this truer than in the ED, with its increasingly high volume of patients. Physicians are under pressure to see patients more and more rapidly, to manage them efficiently, and to maintain a high level of vigilance to identify the few, among many, who have truly emergent needs. The acuity of patients is another major factor in time limitation; just a few critically ill patients may absorb the full attention of the instructor, often for long stretches of time [1].

*Practical Teaching in Emergency Medicine*, 1st edition. Edited by R Rogers, A Mattu, M Winters & J Martinez. ©2009 Blackwell Publishing, ISBN: 9781405176224

At the same time, EDs are being held to more stringent standards of patient satisfaction, meaning that facilitating patient flow and communicating with patients and their families also remains a high priority during a shift. Additional tasks such as directing on-line medical control, receiving calls from primary care physicians and consultants, and arranging inter-hospital transfers contribute to the workload. Emphasis on quality of documentation, out of concern for both billing and litigation, shunts remaining time and energy toward careful charting.

Overall, the demands of patient care leave little time for teaching activities [2]. Unlike other departments in the hospital, the ED cannot set aside structured teaching time as a routine part of the work day in the form of morning report, lunchtime conferences, or extended rounds. Teaching must occur spontaneously and is always subject to interruption, sabotaged by phone calls, incoming traumas, or questions from nurses and other staff [3]. Even without direct interruptions, distraction comes in the form of the ever-present background noise of phones, overhead pages, and voices of staff, patients, and their families. Contributing to the less-than-ideal teaching environment is the limited physical space. Depending on the physical layout of the department, simply finding an open area to gather for teaching can be difficult in an overcrowded ED where hallways are lined with occupied patient gurneys and back-and-forth pedestrian traffic. Discussion about individual cases can be limited further by the lack of privacy.

The makeup of the learner population creates one of the most challenging aspects of teaching in the ED. Learners range from third year medical students to senior emergency medicine trainees to rotators from across medical and surgical disciplines, all with widely divergent skill sets and learning needs [4]. Knowing how to make teaching appropriate for the student being exposed to the ED for the first time, for the ED trainee trying to hone management skills, and for the off-service rotator seeing cases out of their comfort zone requires a subtlety that can seem impossible to achieve within the confines of an 8- or 10-hour shift. Exacerbating this problem is the limited face-to-face time between individual instructors and learners in the ED. In addition, unlike many services in which a learner is paired with a single instructor for an extended and anticipated period, it is a significant challenge to establish any relationship between teacher and learner when there is little longitudinal contact between them.

## Instructor-based obstacles

The barriers to teaching inherent to the ED may exacerbate the personal challenges faced by any medical educator who aims to teach on a daily basis. The ED environment requires a spontaneous and flexible style of teaching that does not come naturally to many people. Training programs do not commonly provide formal education on effective teaching strategies, and young graduates who have recently become attendings may find balancing patient care with the desire to teach extremely challenging. Even experienced physicians may feel uncertain about how best to relate important clinical points. Instructors may interpret the weariness of tired trainees as a lack of interest in learning or may feel intimidated by the niche areas of knowledge owned by off-service rotators. Because teaching is rarely rewarded in concrete ways, instructors may succumb to more explicit pressures to excel in documentation, ED flow, or patient satisfaction, setting aside teaching as a "last priority" that rarely gets attended to.

## Learner-based obstacles

Teachers may have trouble "getting through" to their learners, not because the teachers are ineffective, but the learners themselves encounter obstacles in taking advantage of the educational opportunities of the ED. There are many reasons for resistance to learning. Fatigue may be a factor, especially in non-ED rotators who do not anticipate how demanding an ED schedule can be. In addition, students and trainees may feel overwhelmed by the wide range of clinical entities presenting to the ED and the breadth of clinical tasks they are expected to perform. Some trainees may work in specialty clinic or ambulatory care settings where patients present with a much narrower range of diseases, are generally stable, and are seen and worked up one or two at a time, in serial fashion. Others may believe that their most important duty is to complete the workup of every patient they admit, in order to assist their colleagues on the inpatient wards. All of this may result in learners resisting change – and missing out on the main educational purpose of the ED rotation – by seeking to recreate their comfort zone, selecting out patients with disease entities that are familiar, delaying picking up new patients, or being dismissive of information that they perceive as irrelevant to their ultimate career.

When an educator feels that their instruction is not quite reaching the learner, it may help to stop and consider that (1) the learner may very well inspire this feeling in other ED and non-ED educators, (2) it is unlikely the learner is happy about having this effect, and

(3) it is likely a natural response to stress and uncertainty. These are challenging scenarios but considering some of these factors may prevent frustration and help the instructor ultimately succeed in "getting through."

## Solutions

For the teaching aspirant, the obstacles discussed thus far may seem overwhelming, particularly since many of them – the volume of patients and the number of responsibilities of the attending physician – are likely to only amplify over time. On the bright side, the ED also offers many unique opportunities for teaching, including the wide variety of clinical entities seen, the breadth and the depth of clinical skills practiced, and the constant close contact between instructors and learners during a shift. To take advantage of these strengths, the successful teaching physician will utilize several key teaching strategies (see Box 2.1). Each of these strategies is discussed later.

### Use a wide variety of teaching techniques

The most realistic approach to teaching in the ED is to integrate it with preexisting patient care activities. This requires instructors to be flexible in using a variety of teaching techniques [1, 5, 6]. Preparation and delivery of brief (one or two minute) lecture points can be integrated into any of the dozens of clinical actions performed routinely in the ED – sign-out rounds, patient presentations, interpretation of x-rays or laboratory results, or procedures – ensuring that some level of teaching occurs continuously throughout the shift. Teaching may also occur in the form of feedback, by observing a student or trainee in action and offering reinforcement of things done well and constructive comments on areas needing improvement [7].

Interactive discussion is a simple, effective, and often overlooked teaching technique that can be used to encourage learners

---

**Box 2.1** Strategies for overcoming teaching obstacles in the ED

- Use a wide variety of teaching techniques
- Remember that teaching is a shared responsibility among all members of the clinical staff
- Be prepared for any teaching opportunities that may arise during a shift
- Recognize the importance of *inspiration* as well as *information*
- Spend time outside of clinical shifts acquiring teaching skills

to express what they think and why, to consider alternate possibilities, and to bring up their own areas of uncertainty. Using questions such as "Why do you think that?," "What else could be going on with this patient?," or "What questions do you have?" prompt learners to work through the problem and come up with their own solutions. This process can help instructors get to know individual learners and identify their specific educational goals.

### Remember that teaching is a shared responsibility among all members of the clinical staff

All members of the clinical team should be active partners in the teaching process. Particularly during a busy shift, instructors may acknowledge their own limitations and ask learners to take a greater role in the educational process. Senior trainees can assume responsibility for teaching interns and medical students; trainees at any level can point out interesting cases to others or find articles and other resources to share with their colleagues. Rotators are a potentially rich resource and should be encouraged to share knowledge from the perspective of their specialty training. Nursing staff may also be engaged by contributing to discussion after trauma or medical resuscitations, teaching skills such as intravenous line placement or urinary bladder catheterization or withholding non-emergent patient care issues until the conclusion of a teaching activity.

### Be well prepared for any teaching opportunities that do arise during a shift

Instructors in the ED should be prepared to take advantage of all available opportunities to teach. Despite the "never-know-what's-coming-next" quality of the ED, certain situations occur reliably and lend themselves well to teaching. Sign-out rounds, when all staff are gathered in one place, allow brief discussion of common clinical entities presenting to the ED and are a good opportunity for focused teaching points. High-profile cases such as traumas or resuscitations, which tend to naturally pique the interest of students and trainees, may be followed by a "debriefing" to review core management issues. An unusual presentation or physical finding may be relayed to all learners, even those not directly involved with that patient's care.

While downtime is rare in the ED, it will occasionally occur when the department is well staffed or volume is low. Having a stock activity for unexpected free time will avoid having to teach extemporaneously; a mock code, short lecture, or an easily accessible file of ECGs or radiographs can make even 5 or 10 minutes a high-yield

---

**Box 2.2** Sample educational prescription (Adapted from:
http://www.cebm.utoronto.ca/doc/edupres.doc)

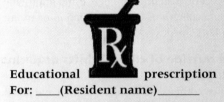

**Educational** **prescription**
**For:** ____(Resident name)_____

**Patient or condition:**

**Clinical question:**

**Date and place to present findings:**

*Presentations will cover:
1. Search strategy;
2. Search results;
3. Validity of the evidence;
4. Importance of the evidence;
5. Applicability of the evidence to your patient.

---

experience. It is also helpful to have a plan for independent learning in case an individual learner has time between patients or while
awaiting for test results; they can be directed to access a teaching file
or find their own resources to review a topic and share it with others by the end of the shift [6, 8]. The use of educational prescription
cards (see sample prescription in Box 2.2) can remind students and
instructors about clinical questions that arise and help to make sure
that they are addressed in a timely fashion.

### Recognize the importance of inspiration as well as information

Often, the actual deficiency faced by the learner will be difficult to
identify. If an intubation has failed because positioning was wrong,
then instruction on adjusting the position can be useful. Yet for the
learner who provides an ineffective oral presentation or seems to miss
the essential clinical observation, the role of educator may be more
inspirational than educational. A supportive word to a struggling

learner emphasizing the learner's abilities and pointing out similar challenges you have encountered in the past (without pointing out that is was when you were a second year medical student) may have far greater impact on instilling confidence and improving performance than providing a solitary piece of information or trying to figure out how to fix an ill-defined weakness.

## Spend time outside of clinical shifts acquiring teaching skills

Teaching, like any other skill, requires training and practice. Outside of the clinical shift, instructors may pursue opportunities to develop their teaching abilities through faculty development seminars and training programs [9–11]. In recent years, the body of literature about effective teaching in the clinical setting [5, 12, 13] – and even specifically in the ED setting (1, 14–16) – has grown tremendously. Compiling and disseminating a faculty curriculum, sharing and reviewing articles in a faculty meeting, or devoting conference time to the discussion of articles can raise awareness of teaching techniques, establish teaching as a high priority in the department, and bypass the relatively, costly alternative of formal faculty development courses.

## Conclusion

With all of the fixed responsibilities of an ED physician, the reminder to add on teaching time that may feel like the proverbial last straw, particularly in a challenging practice environment that contains so many unavoidable obstacles to teaching. However, rich learning potential is also an inherent quality of the ED, and instructors can adopt teaching strategies that will realize this potential, making every shift both educational and inspirational.

---

### Summary points

1. Challenges to teaching arise not only from the busy ED setting itself, but also from instructor- and learner-based factors.
2. Instructors can overcome obstacles to teaching in the ED by using a strategy that incorporates varied teaching techniques, shared teaching responsibility, preparation for spontaneous teaching activities, encouragement of learners, and investment in faculty development programs.
3. Despite many obstacles to teaching, the ED has the potential to be one of the most productive learning environments in the hospital.

# References

1. Atzema C, Bandiera G, Schull MJ. Emergency department crowding: the effect on resident education. *Ann Emerg Med* 2005; 45: 276–281.
2. Chisholm CD, Whenmouth LF, Daly EA, Cordell WH, Giles BK, Brizendine EJ. An evaluation of emergency medicine resident interaction time with faculty in different teaching venues. *Acad Emerg Med* 2004 February; 11(2): 149–155.
3. Chisholm CD, Collison E, Nelson D, Cornell W. Emergency department workplace interruptions: are emergency physicians "interrupt-driven" and "multitasking"? *Acad Emerg Med* 2000; 7: 1239–1243.
4. Carter AJE, McCauley WA. Off-service residents in the emergency department: the need for learner-centeredness. *Can J Emerg Med* 2003; 5(6): 400–405.
5. Furney SL, Orsini A, Orsetti K, *et al*. Teaching the one-minute preceptor. A randomized controlled trial. *J Gen Intern Med* 2001; 16(9): 620–624.
6. Bandiera G, Lee S, Tiberius R. Creating effective learning in today's emergency departments: how accomplished teachers get it done. *Acad Emerg Med* 2005; 45(3): 253–261.
7. Ende J. Feedback in clinical medical education. *JAMA* 1983; 250: 777–781.
8. Pusic MV, Pachev GS, MacDonald WA. Embedding medical student computer tutorials into a busy emergency department. *Acad Emerg Med* 2007; 14(2): 138–148.
9. Bandiera G, Lee S, Foote J. Faculty perceptions and practice impact of a faculty development workshop on emergency medicine teaching. *Can J Emerg Med* 2005; 7(5): 321–327.
10. Berbano EP, Browning R, Pangaro L, Jackson JL. The impact of the Stanford Faculty Development Program on ambulatory teaching behavior. *J Gen Intern Med* 2006; 21 (5): 430–434.
11. Skeff KM, *et al*. The Stanford Faculty Development Program: a dissemination approach to faculty development for medical teachers. *Teach Learn Med* 1992; 4: 174–186.
12. Heidenreich C, Lye P, Simpson D, Lourich M. The search for effective and efficient ambulatory teaching methods through the literature. *Pediatrics* 2000; 105: 231–237.
13. McGee SR, Irby DM. Teaching in the outpatient clinic: practical tips. *J General Int Med* 1997 Apr; 12(Suppl 2): S34–S40.
14. Aldeen AZ, Gisondi MA. Bedside teaching in the emergency department. *Acad Emerg Med* 2006; 13(8): 860–866.
15. Penciner R. Clinical teaching in a busy emergency department: strategies for success. *Can J Emerg Med* 2002; 4(4): 286–288.
16. Richardson BK. Feedback. *Acad Emerg Med* 2004; 11(12): 283: e1–e5.

# CHAPTER 3
# Teaching and patient care in emergency medicine

*Michael A. Bohrn, David A. Kramer*
Department of Emergency Medicine, York Hospital, York, PA, USA

## Introduction

Why do we choose to teach emergency medicine (EM)? This is a question frequently asked of EM faculty. There are a variety of reasons – some obvious and some subtle. Every emergency physician has benefited from the skills of talented educators, role models, and mentors during their career. For some, the chance to give back to future generations is enough motivation. For others, there are external motivators such as teaching awards and the potential for academic promotion. Everyone experiences these motivators to differing degrees, and nearly everyone needs some motivation to make it through challenging times attempting to teach in a busy emergency department (ED). In this chapter, we will explore some of the reasons emergency physicians teach and some of the factors which tie EM teaching to excellence in patient care.

## Motivation for teaching emergency medicine

Faculty teachers in EM choose this profession, and their career roles, for a variety of reasons. For some, it is the simple desire to educate and train future physicians. For others, the personal and career opportunities offered by a career in education make this an

*Practical Teaching in Emergency Medicine*, 1st edition. Edited by R Rogers, A Mattu, M Winters & J Martinez. ©2009 Blackwell Publishing, ISBN: 9781405176224

attractive option. In some specialties, a variety of rewards have been used to stimulate faculty teaching. These include additional financial incentives and educational opportunities, gifts, teaching awards, special recognition events, and appreciation letters [1, 2]. The chance to gain and develop other professional and leadership skills, such as presentation skills, conflict resolution techniques, business communication skills, and project management basics provide a career balance, which helps to maintain motivation and job satisfaction for many educators. In addition, the opportunity to complement an active role in clinical care and teaching with office, educational, and research activities can be a strong motivator.

Tangible motivation for teaching is somewhat less frequently utilized. While many medical schools and institutions now recognize teaching activities and outstanding faculty teachers, internal motivation seems to be more prevalent [2–4]. Similarly, financial incentives for teaching positions usually are not as great as those in private practice [5, 6]. Finally, the opportunity to be a part of, and to interact with, a dynamic teaching faculty within a program, department/division, or institution can be a strong motivator. Associating with colleagues, sharing similar beliefs, goals, and attitudes toward teaching and mentoring residents and students is a key component of the academic environment.

## The beginning educator

Early in an academic career, a medical educator typically focuses on activities related to core medical knowledge. Often, this physician is either preparing for or has recently completed the Board certification exam in EM. This provides fertile ground for teaching activities focusing on core knowledge and skills. Teaching activities early in one's career can also allow development of a variety of administrative skills, including education and curriculum planning, negotiation and communication skills, learning to function amidst organization politics, and time management, and personal development goals. Success in early career activities can set the stage for future leadership positions such as medical student rotation directors, residency program directors, departmental Chairs, and institutional/medical school leadership (e.g. dean's office) positions. Creating and running a successful educational session, class, or program are fundamental steps in faculty development. Transition to future stages of the medical education career carry differing sets of goals, activities, and skills.

## The seasoned veteran

In mid-career, individual goals often change, and educational activities and teaching reflect this. By this point, individual skills, including teaching in one-on-one situations, small groups, and large group sessions have generally developed to a level of proficiency and the focus often shifts to coordination of group educational activities, taking leadership roles for expanding and improving other faculty members' teaching skills, and developing educational curricula and programs. Individual teaching and skills continue to be a focus, but these physicians find themselves to be subject matter experts with regard to medical education and teaching and often seek academic activities, which highlight their unique skills and experiences.

Course directorships and other leadership roles are part of the natural evolution of the medical educator's career during this phase. These physicians have been involved in education long enough to know the basics and understand the common pitfalls to avoid in order to ensure success. They become excellent resources for junior faculty members and can serve as key mentors, collaborators, and role models. Competing administrative, clinical, research, and other interests can change individual career goals, but those interested in continuing a career focusing on medical education develop opportunities to hone specific skills, and might advance toward national and even international prominence.

## The master educator

The next stage of the medical education career often involves publications, speaking engagements, and other high-profile activities. Physicians in this group have the requisite skills and knowledge needed to be effective individual educators but also have gathered the necessary influence and experience to become the true drivers of large-scale medical education activities and curricula. These master educators frequently have time to develop individual educational philosophies and now have the sphere of influence needed to implement and disseminate their ideas.

# The benefits of teaching in emergency medicine

## Training the doctors of tomorrow

Classically deemed the primary goal of academic faculty members, clinical and didactic teaching remains a primary purpose for EM faculty. A major component of the traditional academic "triple threat" of patient care, education, and research, the training of tomorrow's physicians is as important now as it has ever been. With rapid advances in medical technology and informatics, teaching in EM is, in some ways, more challenging as well. Walking the fine line between embracing the technologies of the future while maintaining a bastion of the clinical skills of the past, EM educators are able to provide medical students and physicians-in-training the best of both worlds. In many specialties, physicians proceed directly to test for a multitude of patient presentations. In ED, the initial evaluation of a critically ill or injured patient still boils down to basic clinical skills. In many ways, emergency physicians and educators possess the broadest skill set for the evaluation of acutely ill patients. This benefits medical students, as the ED clerkship is often the first opportunity they have to evaluate undifferentiated acutely ill patients. This unique factor, in addition to the concentration and diversity of patient pathology seen in the typical teaching ED, makes a rotation or training program in EM an outstanding learning experience for physicians-in-training [7].

A natural extension of the key role of EM in medical education is the development of specific rotations in EM. Master educators have led the transformation of these rotations, which continue to become integrated as core components of the undergraduate medical education curriculum [8, 9]. Career development for educators focusing specifically on EM education of undergraduates has led to an appropriate body of knowledge and resources for continued improvements in this area [9, 10].

All of these efforts in undergraduate EM education reflect an increasing responsibility for the preparation of future generations of physicians to provide emergency care. Although some physicians-in-training ultimately will choose careers in academic medicine and teaching, the majority of EM graduates proceed on to careers in non-academic hospital settings [11, 12]. Thus, the teaching provided by the teachers in EM can influence the full spectrum of future academicians as well as community-based physicians. With this broad appeal, EM physicians are sought out to provide guidance for a wide range of future career options.

This role specifically benefits future emergency physicians via a mentoring process. Career guidance, with specific attention to the choice of rotations, schedules, post-graduate training programs, and career goals are all part of the role of the EM educator [13, 14]. There is even a role for virtual advisors (via the internet and E-mail communications) through the Society for Academic Emergency Medicine (SAEM), which allows faculty members to become mentors for students at institutions without EM programs, and for other interested students [15]. Active mentoring occurs on all levels, and mentorship for clinician-educators in EM has also been described [16]. Few other specialties are so invested in the future.

## Developing areas of specialty interest

Within each medical specialty are various areas of subspecialty knowledge and skills, and the field of EM features a wide variety of them. From the formally acknowledged fields of pediatric EM and toxicology, for which subspecialty fellowships have been developed, to a host of other areas – teaching physicians are involved. Emergency ultrasound, administration, emergency medical services (EMS), tactical EMS, medical informatics, international EM, and others have also evolved to include fellowship-training programs and thus require faculty with specific expertise and teaching skills in these areas. Within nearly every academic practice group, various physicians are also known as the "go to" person for questions regarding specific areas. These physicians attain additional knowledge through seminars, mini-fellowships, individual study, and continuing medical education courses, as well as attendance at regional and national meetings such as those sponsored the American Academy of Emergency Medicine (AAEM), the Society for Academic Emergency Medicine (SAEM), and the American College of Emergency Physicians (ACEP). Subject matter experts may have unique skills and knowledge in emergency imaging, domestic violence treatment and education programs, cardiovascular or neurologic emergencies, quality assurance and process improvement activities, medicolegal and risk management processes, geriatric issues, or women's health issues, among others. Medical simulation offers the challenges of integrating medical knowledge, attitudes, and skills in case scenarios, procedure-based learning activities, and role playing, and is emerging as an area of great strength for EM educators [17]. This area should be an important focus for EM education in the future.

With specific educators having advanced knowledge in these areas, opportunities for focused education for medical students and residents abound. In addition, one of the first steps in attaining long-term success in medical research is development of an academic niche or area of expertise. This fosters the generation of research questions and, ultimately, can lead to research studies and other activities. This generation of specialty-specific research has been one of the goals of the specialty of EM since its inception [18, 19].

## Forming the backbone of local, regional, and national organizations

Emergency medicine educators are often leaders in clinical and research activities, as well as leaders within their institutions and communities. Being a part of cutting edge research and patient care activities uniquely positions EM educators to be leaders and participants in a variety of organizations. From an academic standpoint, EM educators interact with students, physicians-in-training, and faculty from nearly every other specialty. This familiarity aids EM educators interested in leadership positions within their departments or divisions and in advancement within the educational and administrative hierarchy of their institution and/or university. From a specialty and political standpoint, the leadership skills gained by interactions within their local institutions, as well as the structured non-clinical time inherent to EM training programs provide opportunities for advancement in regional and national specialty organizations, in addition to medical organizations which cross specialty lines or represent medicine as a whole. Finally, from a community standpoint, the educator in EM often has valuable skills in administration, leadership, and project management. This helps to make them prime candidates for leadership positions within community groups.

## Improving patient care and safety

### Defining the standard of care

The fundamental process of teaching leads to increased critical appraisal of the medical literature and current practices and procedures. Faculty in teaching roles helps to define the standard of practice in EM. A subset of EM practice encompasses procedural skills. Teaching physicians are often innovators of new techniques, approaches, and equipment for procedures. Simulation-based medical education is also an area of intense interest for EM educators [17, 20, 21]. The focus on simulation-based education leads to improved patient care, while applying principles of crew resource management and analysis of medical and systems errors. Educators in EM have also been proactive in designing specific curricula for programs covering patient safety and error reduction [22].

In addition, teaching physicians often are innovators in defining patient care practices, protocols, and procedures which help to define the standard of care in EM. Emergency ultrasound is one such area of keen interest, and innovators in EM education are helping to shape the general medical school curriculum of the future [23]. There is a natural association between research and quality improvement since projects led by EM educators are often linked to changes in patient care. Post-graduate training programs and medical student educational experiences allow interaction between established educators and researchers, and talented new medical professionals. This allows formation of a dynamic organization geared toward producing new knowledge and practices.

## Emergency medicine education: foundations for the future

Perhaps the longest reaching effect of teaching in EM is the joy of seeing students and physicians-in-training from years past succeed and grow to become the next generation of practicing emergency physicians. The role of teacher is not always an easy one, but the benefits are clear. Solid teaching skills and the ability to successfully motivate and involve today's EM learners will result in a stronger, more stable specialty and will positively impact both learners and patients for many years. One high point of EM education lies in the creation of the curriculum guiding all educational activities. The Model of the Clinical Practice of Emergency Medicine represents the hard work of educators, researchers, and administrators in standardizing the goals of EM education [24]. The groups that developed this document, and its recent revisions, include educators who have devoted their careers toward improving EM education and practice for the future [25].

## Conclusion

There are many reasons for teaching EM. Each physician has his specific reasons for participating. Most physicians have several motivators. For many, the desire to be actively involved in clinical, didactic, and research training for tomorrow's emergency physicians appears to be a primary goal. Enhancing patient care and patient safety are common factors, as is the desire to guide and enhance the standards of patient care. Development of specific faculty interest areas, career and professional development, and interaction with a variety of professionals in teaching and administrative roles are significant motivators for some educators. Although the specific reasons for teaching vary from person to person, the overriding goals of advancing our personal and professional lives, and advancing the specialty of EM appeal to all.

## Summary points

1. A variety of educational, business, leadership, and professional development goals shape the career paths of emergency medicine educators.
2. Most educators follow a typical progression en route to the role of Master Educator.
3. Emergency medicine educators have unique opportunities to shape their professional world in the areas of service, leadership, research, and defining standards of care.

## References

1. Kumar A, Loomba D, Rahangdale RY, *et al*. Rewards and incentives for nonsalaried clinical faculty who teach medical students. *J Gen Int Med* 1999; 14: 370–372.
2. Viggiano TR, Shub C, Giere RW. The Mayo Clinic's clinician-educator award: a program to encourage educational innovation and scholarship. *Acad Med* 2000; 75: 940–943.
3. Levinson W, Rubenstein A. Mission-critical: integrating clinician-educators into academic medical centers. *N Engl J Med* 1999; 342: 840–844.
4. Nutter DO, Bond JS, Judith S, *et al*. Measuring faculty efforts and contributions in medical education. *Acad Med* 2000; 75: 199–207.
5. Kristal SL, Randall-Kristal KA, Thompson BM. The Society for Academic Emergency Medicine's 2004–2005 faculty salary and benefit survey. *Acad Emerg Med* 2006; 13: 548–558.
6. MD Salaries. Available at: http://mdsalaries.blogspot.com/2006/05/emergency-medicine-physician-salaries.html. Accessed September 2007.
7. Aldeen AZ, Gisondi MA. Bedside teaching in the emergency department. *Acad Emerg Med* 2006; 13: 860–866.
8. Russi CS, Hamilton GC. A case for emergency medicine in the undergraduate medical school curriculum (commentary). *Acad Emerg Med* 2005; 12: 994–998.
9. Wald DA, Manthey DE, Kruus L, *et al*. The state of the clerkship: a survey of emergency medicine clerkship directors. *Acad Emerg Med* 2007; 14: 629–634.

10. Coates WC. An educator's guide to teaching EM to medical students. *Acad Emerg Med* 2004; 11: 300–306.

11. Lubavin BV, Langdorf MI, Blasko BJ. The effect of emergency medicine residency format on pursuit of fellowship training and academic career. *Acad Emerg Med* 2004; 11: 938–943.

12. Stern SA, Hyungjin MK, Neacy K, *et al.* The impact of environmental factors on emergency medicine resident career choice. *Acad Emerg Med* 1999; 6: 262–270.

13. Coates WC, Hobgood CD, Birnbaum A, *et al. Faculty development*: academic opportunities for emergency medicine faculty on education career tracks. *Acad Emerg Med* 2003; 10: 1113–1117.

14. Garmel GM. Mentoring medical students in academic emergency medicine. *Acad Emerg Med* 2004; 11: 1351–1357.

15. Coates WC, Ankel F, Birnbaum A, *et al.* The Virtual Advisor Program: linking students to mentors via the World Wide Web. *Acad Emerg Med* 2004; 11: 253–255.

16. Farrell SE, Digioia NM, Broderick KB, *et al.* Mentoring for clinician–educators. *Acad Emerg Med* 2004; 11: 1346–1350.

17. Bond WF, Lammers RL, Spillane LL, *et al.* The use of simulation in emergency medicine: a research agenda. *Acad Emerg Med* 2007; 14: 353–363.

18. Biros MH, Barsan WG, Lewis RJ, *et al.* Supporting emergency medicine research: developing the infrastructure. *Ann Emerg Med* 1998; 31: 188–196.

19. Pollack CV, Cairns CB. The Emergency Medicine Foundation: 25 years of advancing education and research. *Ann Emerg Med* 1999; 33: 448–450.

20. Binstadt ES, Walls RM, White BA, *et al.* A comprehensive medical simulation education curriculum for emergency medicine residents. *Ann Emerg Med* 2007; 49: 505–507.

21. McFetrich J. A structured literature review on the use of high fidelity simulators for teaching emergency medicine. *Emerg Med J* 2006; 23: 509–511.

22. Croskerry P, Wears RL, Binder LS, *et al.* Setting the educational agenda and curriculum for error prevention in emergency medicine. *Acad Emerg Med* 2007; 7: 1194–1200.

23. Cook T, Hunt P, Hoppman R. Emergency medicine leads the way for training students in clinician-based ultrasound: a radical paradigm shift in patient imaging. *Acad Emerg Med* 2007; 14: 558–561.

24. Hockberger RS, La Duca A, Orr NA, *et al.* Creating the model of the clinical practice of emergency medicine: the case of emergency medicine. *Acad Emerg Med* 2003; 10: 161–168.

25. Thomas HA, Binder LS, Chapman DM, *et al.* The 2003 model of the clinical practice of emergency medicine: the 2005 update. *Acad Emerg Med* 2006; 13: 1070–1073.

## SECTION 2
# Teaching in the Emergency Department

# CHAPTER 4

# Bedside teaching in the emergency department

*Kevin G. Rodgers*
Professor of Clinical Emergency Medicine, Co-Program Director, Emergency Medicine
Residency, Indiana University School of Medicine, Indianapolis, IN, USA

*A picture is worth a thousand words!*
FRED R. BARNARD'S CHINESE PROVERB

*Medicine is learned at the bedside and not in the classroom; the best
teaching is that taught by the patient himself.*
SIR WILLIAM OSLER

Emergency medicine (EM) faculty have the optimal opportunity
to teach at the patient bedside on a daily basis. Although typically
focused on trainee and medical student education, the audience
may also include nurses and ancillary personnel as well as patients
and their families. Regardless of the target, the teaching concepts
are the same: Be enthusiastic, focus on the learner's needs, and
give a concise, clear, focused message.

Bedside teaching is not a new idea. Over twenty centuries ago
Hippocrates stepped out of the classroom (actually it was the temple) to practice medicine at the bedside based on the value of direct
observation. Sir William Osler, the father of modern day bedside
teaching, felt that bedside instruction was the best environment for
physician education [1].

Indeed, the emergency department (ED) is possibly the most fertile ground for bedside teaching in medicine. Twenty-four hours a
day it consistently provides unlimited opportunities to see undifferentiated patients with a diversity of disease processes that
cross all subspecialties of medicine and all socioeconomic groups.
Emergency physicians (EP) also have the prospect of interacting
with not only a variety of physicians at different levels of training,

*Practical Teaching in Emergency Medicine*, 1st edition. Edited by R Rogers, A Mattu,
M Winters & J Martinez. ©2009 Blackwell Publishing, ISBN: 9781405176224

but also virtually the entire scope of the health care team. Yet most EP are experiencing intense pressure to improve the efficiency, documentation, and cost effectiveness of EM practice. These specific external pressures inherent to EM combined with other well-known barriers that all clinician-educators face, has resulted in a significant decline in the amount and the quality of bedside teaching. Time spent at the bedside teaching and observing resident skills has dwindled from 75% 30 years ago to 15–20% or less today [2].

## What's holding us back: barriers to bedside teaching

Classically, bedside teaching occurred on inpatient ward rounds conducted by academic professors in university teaching hospitals. This environment was a stable one where patient centered teaching could be conducted at a calculated pace without interruptions. Unfortunately, in recent years modern medical education has come to embrace a more didactic-based format at the expense of bedside teaching due to a variety of reasons [3, 4]. Lecture-based curricula are a more easily implemented "passive approach" that requires fewer instructors, less work ethic, and no expectation for "bedside teaching skills." This didactic approach alleviates instructor's concerns over the need for an "expert performance" at the bedside and eliminates any unwanted involvement of the patient in discussions about their own care, so called medical chauvinism. The academic community itself has contributed to this migration by failing to provide faculty development in the critical skill set needed for successful bedside teaching as well as under-appreciating the "value" of accomplished clinician-teachers with regard to promotion and financial support [5, 6]. Finally, time constraints in the ED associated with efficient and effective patient management, exert a negative influence on the time spent at the bedside.

Educators can easily overcome these obstacles with some enthusiasm, a little training, a realization that experts can say, "I don't know" and a commitment to improving health care in general. Bedside teaching improves everyone it touches, including the patient, even if they are not the intended target. The overwhelming majority of patients feel educated and reassured about their illness and their diagnostic and therapeutic plan and have a better opportunity to get their questions answered. The impact of direct observation during bedside encounters cannot be understated. Direct observation can positively affect not only history and physical examination skills, but procedural ability, professionalism, interpersonal skills, and communication as well [7, 8]. Linking teaching with a visual cue (the patient) is very powerful tool that can impact the quality of care provided by the entire health care team. Successful bedside teaching does require some planning and utilization of several attributes and skills that anyone can develop.

## The basics: characteristics of effective bedside teachers

Until a study published by Bandiera *et al.* [9] in 2005, research supporting characteristics for effective bedside teaching in the ED were primarily adapted from other practice environments. Personality characteristics describing the best teachers are well known: enthusiastic, available, knowledgeable, confident, receptive, inquisitive (Table 4.1). Unfortunately, personality alone does not guarantee learner success. Heidenreich [10] and Bandiera both examined effective and efficient strategies for teaching in the ambulatory and ED settings respectively (Table 4.2). A combination of the right personality traits and some easily learned and implemented learning strategies result in successful bedside teaching.

Success begins with enthusiasm and a desire to positively influence the learner. Excellent teachers seek opportunities to teach and share cases even with learners they are not supervising. They plan ahead, developing and utilizing additional teaching resources to augment their clinical-based instruction. This may include case files; electronic depositories of clinical photos, radiographs, EKGs, research articles or handouts; or web-based teaching sites. They

**Table 4.1** Characteristics of excellent bedside teachers [9, 10].

- Enthusiastic
- Available, approachable, patient, calm, respectful, tolerates errors
- Excellent listener
- Knowledgeable but realistic and willing to say "I don't know, let's find out"
- Actively seeks opportunities to teach
- Role model for professionalism, communication, and interpersonal skills, life-long learning
- Effective, efficient and timely

**Table 4.2** Strategies for effective ED teaching [9, 10].

---

- Orients the learner by relaying clearly defined expectations of their performance

- Optimizes faculty–learner interaction using optimal interpersonal skills and teaching tools such as the Internet, teaching files, prepared cases

- Provides a clear, concise, focused message ("teaching bite") and avoids "over-teaching"

- Provides learner centered instruction with instruction prioritized and tailored to the learner's needs

- Promotes learner autonomy and facilitates active problem-solving and critical thinking skills through teacher–learner reflection

- Teaches in the patient's presence and mentors and reinforces effective behaviors (reflective modeling)

- Demonstrates with clarity examination and procedural skills

- Improves the environment – insures adequate time to teach without interruptions

- Provides effective, prompt feedback

---

employ and mentor effective interpersonal and communication skills to establish a receptive learning environment. This includes projecting a supportive, approachable, calm demeanor.

As the shift begins, get to know the learner and ascertain their educational needs and focus for the shift. Learner centered instruction was the single most commonly cited effective learning strategy by EM educators [9]. Relay upfront clear expectations for learner performance. Foster a collegial atmosphere that encourages an open exchange of ideas. This requires being an active listener; teachers should listen more and talk less. Ask questions which promote learner autonomy, critical thinking, problem-solving, and linking of new elements to the learners' existing fund of knowledge. Ask the learners to commit to their ideas and allow them to make mistakes; this provides an excellent framework for discussion and feedback. Allow time and opportunity for self-assessment and reflection of the learner. Be knowledgeable but realistic and willing to say "I don't know, let's find out." Teach how to search for the best evidence and apply it to patient care in real time (knowledge translation). This is a critical facet of mentoring life-long learning.

Recognize and seize the teachable moment; every case can provide a teaching point. Be creative. When faced with a clinically common or unchallenging case, change the age, alter the setting to a community hospital with fewer resources, or throw in a hypothetical "curve-ball" lab or clinical finding. Provide a clear, concise, focused message ("teaching bite") delivered at the learner's level that insures their reception. Avoid "over-teaching" or providing an excessive amount of information that obscures or clutters the intended teaching point. If you provide more than one teaching point, provide a summary at the end of your discussion.

Unfortunately, even the most enthusiastic, skilled, well-intentioned teachers are often thwarted in their efforts by "environmental issues." Frequent interruptions, a full waiting room and competing demands on a busy clinical shift all conspire to negate effective learning. Sometimes just finding a quiet place to discuss a case is nearly impossible. Academic faculty must proactively "design" an environment conducive to learning. This begins by insuring faculty and departmental buy-in by including the provision of quality education in the department's mission statement. Thus implementation of "solutions" is supported by a collective mandate. Many academic EM departments utilize the "teach-only" attending approach whereby one faculty's sole purpose on each shift is to teach and evaluate [8]. Others employ "uninterrupted teaching rounds" where they share teaching points from all the patients in the ED at the beginning or end of each shift with only critical interruptions from the ED staff allowed. Most departments have purposely designed "team areas" where cases can be discussed while maintaining patient privacy. Ultimately the best place for teaching to take place is still at the bedside!

## The framework: the experience versus explanation cycle

Enthusiasm and interactive educational skills that enhance active learning and aid the learner in developing critical thinking skills is only half the battle. Cox has noted that bedside teaching also requires developing a framework in advance that the educational experience will follow. This framework can be divided into two connected cycles starting at the bedside with the experience cycle and followed by the explanation cycle [11, 12]. The "experience cycle" includes the preparation, briefing, clinical experience, and debriefing phases.

Preparation begins with determination of the needs of both the teacher and the learner and communicates expectations for the educational encounter. Teachers must recognize the inherent limitations and set appropriate, limited goals for each encounter. Prior to starting the experience cycle, answer the simple question: what would everyone like to accomplish? This is also the phase during which resources are identified and developed (classic articles, websites, PDA resources, departmental intranet teaching files).

The "briefing phase" prepares both the patient and the learner for the clinical encounter. It consists of an introduction and an explanation of the purpose of the bedside encounter, a discussion of the ground rules with the learner, and a review of any potential examinations or procedures that may be performed. The actual "clinical encounter" provides an excellent opportunity to mentor the performance of the history and the physical examination, demonstrate physical examination findings and procedures, model patient interaction skills, guide and develop critical thinking skills, and provide feedback. As learners become more advanced in their clinical experience and skill set, teachers by design should allow the learner more autonomy and responsibility with regard to diagnostic and therapeutic decision-making. The hallmark of an excellent teacher is allowing the exact right amount of learner autonomy while covertly observing patient care to prevent medical error.

The bedside encounter is also a superb opportunity to enlighten patients about their disease process. It provides a chance to explain what testing and therapeutics will occur and to reinforce and educate about your plans for treatment and follow-up after discharge. The experience cycle ends with the "debriefing phase" which allows the learner an opportunity to answer any "sensitive questions" not raised in front of the patient. The teacher then reviews what was learned at the bedside, insures that the learner received the correct learning points and provides constructive feedback and devises plans for future encounters.

The "explanation cycle" begins with reflection and is followed by explication, working knowledge, and preparation for future patients. Reflection allows the teacher and the student to link practice with theory and previous experiences or knowledge whereas explication examines how medical practice can be improved by advances in biomedical science or current best evidence (practice-based learning). This links the clinical experience with theory and research relevant to the case and brings evidence-based medicine to the bedside by providing an opportunity to assign clinical questions that the learners can use to develop their life-long learning skills and spark future, off line learning. The explanation cycle concludes with the "working knowledge" phase which derives and solidifies practical knowledge from the clinical experience that can be applied to future encounters.

Another popular framework employed to guide bedside teaching is the five-step microskills model of clinical teaching [13]. In a hectic ED, this model provides a condensed version of the aforementioned experience–explanation cycle model and incorporates many of the effective learning strategies identified by Bandiera [9]. The basic steps are (1) Get a commitment, (2) Probe for supporting evidence, (3) Discuss a teaching pearl, (4) Reinforce what was done right (5) Correct mistakes. These will be discussed in other chapters.

## Implementation: the art of bedside questioning

Bedside teaching should be an interactive session that maintains **active** learner participation. Passive learning occurs when teachers talk too much, ask close-ended questions, or answer their own questions. Passive learning is not only ineffective and inefficient, but the learners are also often perceived as disinterested (and it's the teacher's fault!). Envision yourself as a coach and a facilitator that promotes critical thinking by the student. Teaching critical thinking skills will have more of a lasting impact on learners than other methods, like "pimping" (asking learners obscure medical questions to see how much they know or do not know). When skillfully asked, questions should assist the learners in identifying relationships and linking the unknown to the known. Formulate questions that provide the stimulus for the teacher and the student to explore ideas and solutions together. Expert clinical teachers employ guiding questions to focus the learner, promote understanding, probe their reasoning, crystallize an idea or challenge (without confrontation) a conclusion (Table 4.3) [14]. These questions focus on synthesis and interpretation of knowledge as opposed to a simple recall of facts.

Clearly the "style" in which questions are asked has tremendous impact on the learner's perception of a positive or a negative learning climate. Questions that are unexpected, confrontational, accusatory, or used to make a student feel bad create a negative environment and hinder learning. This is also true of teachers who

**Table 4.3** High yield questions (focus, probe, prompt, challenge) [11].

---

- Why do you believe that to be true?
- What have you learned so far?
- How did you reach that conclusion?
- What is your reasoning behind that question?
- What led you to that decision?
- What are some other possibilities that would explain that presentation?
- Why is that information important?
- Why is one approach better than another, are there other approaches we have not considered?
- What will happen if you do/don't do X or Y?
- What is the association between those two findings?

---

exhibit negative body language, ask "rapid-fire" questions, or continually interrupt their student's answers.

In contradistinction, the teacher who seeks to develop critical thinking and successful learning asks meaningful, probing questions in a nonthreatening, positive climate. Their questions stimulate and challenge the learner to analyze, to solve problem, and think independently [15]. This interactive collegial discussion should be immediately followed by formative feedback. Adjectives applied to effective formative feedback include timely, relevant, descriptive, verifiable, focused, and constructive. It should include both positive and negative reinforcement best delivered as the "Sackett Sandwich" (positive–negative–positive). Finally, the "art" of questioning allows teachers to convey their interests, inject their enthusiasm, and continue their own life-long learning.

As teachers, the types of questions we ask also determine the level of intellectual challenge for the learner. Convergent or close-ended questions require little critical thinking whereas probing questions require independent assessment, critical analysis, and problem-solving skills. A blend of convergent, divergent, and probing questions will help keep bedside teaching an active, challenging process. On the average, instructors will only wait two to three seconds after a question before answering it themselves. Studies have shown that the optimal wait-time is actually 17 seconds.

Although this seems like an eternity, teachers must recognize variables which influence expert–novice interactions.

Be cognizant of the fact that expert and novice thought processes take very different pathways through the brain. Experts jump from A→E quickly with little conscious thought process in-between; novices think more concretely in a step-wise A→B→ C→D→E process that is much slower. For this reason, experts who have long forgotten the drawn out step-wise links, have a difficult time explaining their thought process and conclusions to novices. Consider the following descriptors which illustrate the novice versus expert thought process.

| Novice | | Expert |
|---|---|---|
| Sparse | **Knowledge of Subject** | Detailed |
| Limited | **Experience** | Extensive |
| Slow | **Pattern Recognition** | Rapid |
| Isolated Facts | **Memory** | Concepts |

Experts in bedside teaching recognize this processing gap and take the time to explain their thought process and decision-making in a step-wise, point-to-point fashion [16].

## Closure: effective feedback as it relates to bedside teaching

The bedside experience should end with effective, formative feedback. Many researchers have proven that consistent, objective, and timely feedback on performance is the educational intervention most likely to produce a meaningful change in the behavior of professional trainees [17]. Yet, errors are repeated 70% of the time after feedback is provided. Students have poor recall of the "corrective" message in post-encounter feedback. Feedback is rarely provided to physicians-in-training, nurses, or pre-hospital care providers: less than 10% of student/resident patient interactions are followed by feedback and less than 20 seconds of the average 4 minute "teaching" encounter in clinical settings is formative feedback [18]. Finally, students and faculty have different perceptions about what should be included in feedback.

Feedback is the backbone of formative evaluation and should occur continually in clinical teaching. It is real-time "coaching" that occurs in the immediate proximity of the action or behavior being observed. When delivered correctly, it is the most effective tool for reinforcing good behaviors and extinguishing negative ones. This sounds so easy and straightforward, how do we fail?

Unfortunately, first and foremost, teachers were never taught how to give effective feedback. Commonly the feedback lacked a vital component thus rendering it ineffective. Criteria used to define effective feedback include its objectivity, consistency, timeliness, relevance, and clarity. It should be descriptive, verifiable, and focused enough to have a defined impact on the learner. (Table 4.4)

The method of delivering feedback may have been flawed and thus it went unheard. Giving feedback is an interpersonal skill. It requires five key ingredients from the teacher: caring, trust, acceptance, openness, and concern. Feedback presented in this manner minimizes defensiveness and maximizes the learner's ability to change behaviors. Feedback that is poorly defined or cluttered is also often missed.

If the behavioral objectives were ill-defined, then it is difficult to give focused, meaningful feedback. Behavioral expectations must be identified ahead of time so that the learner clearly understands what behaviors the teacher is observing. This provides the basis for descriptive feedback that is focused and specific enough to reinforce positive and alter negative behaviors.

**Table 4.4** Feedback tips.

- Allow for self-evaluation initially

- Raise issues with questions instead of telling

- Do not overwhelm with information (1 message = 75% retention; 2 = 50%; 3 = 25%)

- Do not personalize the message – focus on changing behaviors: avoid inflammatory language; use neutral language; use the collective "we"

- Structure feedback as an ego or "Sackett" sandwich

  – Praise learner for appropriate responses or procedures done well

  – Identify performance problems and correct

  – Finish conversation with positive or encouraging overall summary

- Remember the 4 P's – **Praise in Public...Perfect in Private**

- Use focused, concrete feedback...give your reasoning not just the answer

- Ask student to summarize "take-home messages" from feedback

Faculty may be hesitant to provide constructive criticism because they fear loss of camaraderie or unwarranted negative assessment of their teaching capabilities because they provided critical but honest feedback. They may also withhold feedback because they want the learner to initiate self-assessment, or because they are worried about hurting the learner's self-esteem. A classic problem in the ED, where a learner may interact with multiple teachers in the same shift, is the assumption by one faculty that the negative behavior only occurred during their interaction with the student, or that another faculty was going to provide the formative feedback. In either account, an opportunity to modify behavior is missed and the inappropriate action continues unimpeded.

Thus, the first step in developing constructive feedback is defining expectations or the observable standards of performance that are realistic and clearly communicated to the learners. Next, the teachers must determine learner performance based on focused, objective measures. The best method of evaluation is direct observation at the bedside using a tool such as the Council of Residency Directors (CORD) Standardized Direct Observation Assessment Tool [8]. Other methods that are less reliable include Objective Structured Clinical Examinations (OSCEs), anecdotal report from other teachers, self-report by the student, indirect assessment, and written examinations. The third and potentially most important aspect of providing effective feedback is identification of causes of substandard performance. Without this knowledge, it is virtually impossible for the teacher to design a plan for remediation that will improve the learner's performance. Common causes of substandard performance include a skill or behavior that was never learned or learned incorrectly, skill deterioration from lack of use (e.g. "rusty"), lack of incentive (e.g. student's perception of effort versus likely reward), or environmental issues (e.g. clinic operation hinders student performance). Once identified, the teacher can intervene by providing focused feedback alone, feedback and a refresher, more practice or extensive retraining (remediation).

## Summary

Every case has a teaching point and potentially dozen of "teaching moments." Taking advantage of these opportunities requires the close attention of the teacher to "seize the moment." By employing the aforementioned skills and attributes of successful teachers in an enthusiastic and an efficient manner, EM clinician-educators can have a dramatic impact on a variety of learners. Search out the "teaching moment." Have a number of "teaching bites" and other resources readily available to use when such moments arise. Make sure that your "teaching bite" is focused, easily digestible, and targeted to the learners' level of understanding and their needs. Learn to recognize your learner's knowledge gaps and exploit them for teaching. Guide learning with high yield questions that require synthesis and interpretation. Provide clear, constructive feedback that reinforces the appropriate performance and extinguishes the negative. Most of all enjoy the opportunity to learn from your students/trainees at the bedside as much as they learn from you.

## Summary points

1. **Barriers** to bedside teaching include frequent interruptions, time constraints, and the perceived lack of "value" assigned to teaching by promotions committees.
2. **Basics** of successful teachers include being enthusiastic and prepared, learner centered, and willing to "seize the teachable moment."
3. **Framework** of teaching includes the experience and explanation cycles.
   a. Experience cycle:  *Preparation* – what do you want to accomplish?
   *Briefing* – Introduction, explanation of purpose, ground rules, review of any examinations or procedures to be performed
   *Clinical encounter* – the actual patient encounter
   *Debriefing* after the encounter
   b. Explanation:  *Reflection* – on theory and previous encounters
   *Explication* – how practice can be improved through evidence-based medicine
   *Working knowledge* – deriving knowledge to be applied to future encounters
4. **Implement** your program through active learner participation to *focus* the learner, *promote* understanding, *probe* their reasoning, *crystallize* an idea, and *challenge* their conclusion.
5. **Close** the session by giving effective, prompt feedback.

# References

1. Thayer WS. Osler the teacher. *Bull Johns Hopkins Hosp* 1919; 30: 198–200. 1980; 303: 1230–1233.
2. Collins GF, Cassie JM, Daggett CJ. The role of the attending physician in clinical training. *J Med Educ* 1978; 53: 429–431.
3. Ramani S, Orlander JD, Strunun L, Barber TW. Whither bedside teaching? A focus-group study of clinical teachers. *Acad Med* 2003; 78: 384–390.
4. Ahmed M El. What is happening to bedside teaching? *Med Educ* 2002; 36: 1185–1188.
5. Porter DD. Call for a recommitment to clinical teaching. *Acad Med* 2001; 76: 1114–1115.
6. Stites S, Vansaghi L, Pingleton S, *et al.* Aligning compensation with education: design and implementation of the educational value unit (EVU) system in an academic internal medicine department. *Acad Med* 2005; 80: 1100–1106.
7. Accreditation Council for Graduate Medical Education. Outcome Project. Available at: http://www.acgme.org/Outcome. Assessed November 20, 2007.
8. Shayne P, Gallahue F, Rinnert S, *et al.* on behalf of the CORD SDOT Study Group. Reliability of a Core Competency Checklist assessment in the Emergency Department: the Standardized Direct Observation Assessment Tool. *Acad Emerg Med* 2006; 13: 727–732.
9. Bandiera G, Lee S, Tiberius R. Creating effective learning in today's emergency departments: how accomplished teachers get it done. *Ann Emerg Med* 2005; 45: 253–261.
10. Heidenreich C, Lye P, Simpson D, Lourich M. The search for effective and efficient ambulatory teaching methods through the literature. *Pediatrics* 2000; 105: 231–237.
11. Hayden, SR. Developing a career in the scholarship of teaching as a clinician-educator. In The SAEM/AACEM Faculty Development Handbook. Found at www.saem.org/facdev. Assessed November 20, 2007.
12. Cox K. Planning bedside teaching – 1. Overview. *Med J Aust* 1993; 158: 280–282.
13. Neher JO, Gordon KC, Meyer B, *et al.* A five-step "microskills" model of clinical teaching. *J Am Board Fam Pract* 1992; 5: 419–424.
14. Henderson W. Bedside questioning to promote critical thinking: the art of teaching without pimping. Handout from: EMF/ACEP Teaching Fellowship. 1990.
15. Walker SE. Active learning strategies to promote critical thinking. *J Athl Train* 2003; 38: 263–267.
16. Bransford JD, Brown AL, Cocking RR. *How People Learn: Brain, Mind, Experience, and School.* The National Academies Press, Washington, 1999.
17. Ende J. Feedback in clinical medical education. *JAMA* 1982; 250: 777–781.
18. Irby DM. Teaching and learning in ambulatory care settings: a thematic review of the literature. *Acad Med* 1995; 70: 898–931.

# CHAPTER 5

# Teaching procedures: beyond "see one, do one, teach one"

*Mercedes Torres, Siamak Moayedi*
*University of Maryland, School of Medicine, Baltimore, MD, USA*

## Introduction

Teaching medical procedures may be one of the most rewarding aspects of medical education. Indeed, physicians-in-training place a high value on mastering clinical procedures and often link their confidence to procedural skills. Traditionally, physicians have learned to perform medical procedures by the "see one, do one, teach one" method where a learner observes a procedure, performs one under supervision, and then is considered sufficiently skilled to teach it to others. Furthermore, the majority of such procedures are taught by junior and senior level trainees who may not have mastered their technical or teaching skills. There are inherent flaws to this approach of procedural education. The purpose of this chapter is to provide the necessary theory-based framework for successfully and efficiently teaching psychomotor skills in the emergency department (ED).

## Prepare to teach and learn

Prior to instructing anyone in the performance of a procedure, it is important to provide an opportunity for the student to prepare to learn that procedure. This phase of learning should occur in a

*Practical Teaching in Emergency Medicine*, 1st edition. Edited by R Rogers, A Mattu, M Winters & J Martinez. ©2009 Blackwell Publishing, ISBN: 9781405176224

more didactic format, aside from the lab or patient bedside where the actual mechanics of the procedure will be performed. The goal of this preparatory time is to ensure that they understand the large amount of prerequisite information needed to perform procedures appropriately. This information includes a review of the indications and the contraindications for the procedure, the instruments and the tools used to perform the procedure, and the expected outcome of the procedure. In addition, the learner should take time to review the risks of any procedure they perform, including the possible complications and how to manage those complications if they were to occur. A portion of this preparation should focus on the process of obtaining informed consent as well as the documentation of the procedure itself [1, 2].

Whether procedural instruction is a planned activity (e.g. as a cadaver/skills lab or simulation session) or an impromptu bedside opportunity, the learner should be asked to prepare by acquiring information regarding the procedure prior to its performance. There are several methods instructors can use to prepare students for procedural learning. Traditionally, learners have been assigned chapters in a textbook to review prior to an instructional session or an expected rotation where that procedure is frequently performed. Other approaches include distribution of information packets, computer programs, or videos containing the information they would like the learner to have mastered prior to the teaching experience. Although these methods of preparation will ultimately provide the learner with the information required, they are forms of passive learning. Rather than providing all of this background information directly, instructors can foster interest and more sustained learning if they provide students the tools needed to find this information through their own exploration. Physicians-in-training are often able to uncover and retain more information if they consult multiple sources, including colleagues, texts, nurses, and web-based media. The prospect of learning and performing a new procedure typically serves as adequate motivation for this active learning to occur. In this case, the instructor's role is to provide some guidance regarding sources of reliable information and to review the information acquired, leading a discussion regarding what they have learned and highlighting key points. Even when a bedside procedural teaching opportunity arises with little warning, as long as time permits for patient safety, the student can be directed to take a few minutes to review the key components and details of the procedure in a text or video prior to participating in the tactile learning experience. The teacher should maintain an online or readily accessible repository of videos and texts of common procedures for quick reference in these cases [1].

Although students prepare to learn a procedure, the instructor must also be prepared to teach. This will involve a skill known as task analysis, where the instructor breaks down the procedure into small, more digestible components for teaching purposes. For example, when teaching placement of a central line, one of the micro skills that needs to be acquired prior to attempting the procedure as a whole is the skill of drawing back on a syringe in a single-handed method. Without accomplishing this smaller component of the motor skill, the physician will never successfully learn to place a central line independently. As this example demonstrates, instructor preparation can be challenging as many of the micro skills required to perform procedures are taken for granted once the procedure is mastered. Therefore, instructors must take the time to deconstruct the components of the procedure in preparation for the learning session and create a task analysis. They should develop a clear and concise order for the process being taught in digestible steps, without taking any previous knowledge or experience for granted [3, 4].

The final component of instructor preparation involves the learning environment itself. Maximization of the learning experience is highly dependent upon the setting. As such, when planning to provide procedural instruction at the bedside, instructors must take the time to prepare not only the learner, but the subject as well. For bedside learning on awake and alert patients this step is imperative. In addition to informing the patient that there will be a less-experienced trainee involved in the procedure, it is wise to advise the patient that the procedure will be closely supervised by an experienced teacher and that instructional discussion will be occurring during the procedure. This provides the optimal situation where the patient is not surprised or apprehensive when instruction is being provided during the procedure. In addition, preparing the patient allows for selection of patients who seem more receptive to participating in the learning environment, therefore creating a positive teaching experience for all involved [1].

When the procedural experience involves cadaveric or nonhuman subjects, this phase of the preparation should focus on ensuring that the physical space and the environment is conducive to the type of teaching which is planned. Furthermore, attention is required to ensure the safety of the procedure with respect to communicable disease and proper disposal of sharp medical tools and biologic materials. Finally, care must be taken to ensure that there is an adequate instructor-to-student ratio. Ideally, there will be less than four learners per instructor. In addition, it is imperative that the learners are at the same level of experience to ensure an appropriate and a consistent amount of guidance is provided.

## The process of learning

Although a variety of methods are used for procedural instruction, a process that is based on the theory of psychomotor learning is often most effective. The long standing tenet "see one, do one, teach one" does not provide an optimal framework for the learner or the instructor to ensure mastery of a procedure. Instead, a multistep process of learning performance and then practicing it with a declining level of supervision and guidance is more effective (Table 5.1). This process starts with conceptualization of the procedure, which entails understanding the reasons for performing the procedure as well as the risks and benefits, as described earlier in this chapter. Once conceptualization has occurred, the subsequent step is visualization of the procedure. As the instructor models the procedure in its entirety, the learner is a silent observer, taking mental notes of the instructor's actions. The instructor serves as a silent model during this step of the learning process, demonstrating the expected performance once skill mastery is achieved. Visualization can occur at the bedside, in the cadaver lab, or using previously filmed videos.

**Table 5.1** Steps in the process of learning a procedure.

---

1 *Conceptualization* – understanding the reasons for performing a given procedure, the overall process, the tools involved, and the risks/benefits.

2 *Visualization* – observing a demonstration of the procedure, performed in a fluid and competent fashion by the master teacher.

3 Verbalization – reviewing a verbal deconstruction of the procedure while it is performed by the expert, with opportunity for interruptions and clarifications.

4 *Guided practice* – attempting to perform sequential steps of the procedure under the supervision of an expert physician.

---

It is important to ensure that the learner is positioned to observe the procedure from the same perspective which they will perform the procedure. For example, placing the learner at the patient's side to observe an endotracheal intubation would be suboptimal. Rather, the learner should be positioned with the same visual orientation as the person performing the procedure in relation to the patient, to visually record each step from the perspective in which it is performed.

Once the basis for the procedure is understood (conceptualization) and the learner has been provided with a model of the procedure (visualization), the instructor deconstructs the procedure for the student while performing it a second time, verbally noting each step taken and the skills required for performance of the step. This process is known as verbalization. Accurate task analysis prior to the instructional session ensures that the instructor presents the procedure in a clear, coherent, and comprehensible manner. Each particular portion of the procedure is verbally described as well as physically performed simultaneously. This can be accomplished in a face-to-face interaction or using video prepared in advance. During this step, the learner is encouraged to interrupt the procedure to ask questions or make clarifications of the information being communicated. Although a prepared video may allow for demonstration of the procedure with verbal cues, the interactive discussion regarding particular components of the procedure is best accomplished in a small group or individual, face-to-face interaction. Subsequently, the learner can be asked to provide the verbal narration of the procedure while the instructor performs the procedure a second time. This ensures that the learner conceptually understands the actions involved and the order in which they should be performed [2, 5].

Although multiple faculty members may be involved in teaching procedural skills to the same group of learners, at the bedside as well as in a simulation or cadaver lab, it is of utmost importance that the procedure is consistently demonstrated and performed. Although clinicians who have mastered clinical procedures often have their own nuances or specific tricks of the trade to offer trainees, these should not be incorporated into this stage of the learning process. Therefore, it is important to be cognizant of the basics of a procedure, as some instructors may have to alter their "usual" method for performing a procedure to allow a more standardized educational experience. Once the standard method is mastered by the learner, particular variations and short-cuts may be taught, but if taught prematurely these will only serve to confuse the novice learner and lengthen the time required for motor learning of the procedure [3].

Armed with the visual model of the procedure and the ability to verbalize the steps involved, the learner is then observed attempting to physically perform the procedure on the model. This process is known as guided practice [3]. To decrease learner anxiety, this step is often initially performed on cadavers, simulation models, or a willing volunteer, rather than a patient. The learner may be instructed regarding separate steps of the procedure in a piecemeal fashion, or may attempt the entire procedure under guidance. If the instructor chooses to review certain steps of the procedure, they should be reviewed in the order in which they are performed to maximize the motor-based learning involved. The learner should be able to verbalize each step as they perform it, and should be observed carefully by the instructor for any errors [3].

When an error is identified, it is optimal to have the instructor place their hand on the hand of the trainee to stop the incorrect action and physically redirect them to the correct motor action while providing verbal instruction regarding the proper method. It is important that the learner is told that this will happen and for them to expect this hand-on-hand contact. One common pitfall is allowing learners to perform procedures with errors and then providing feedback regarding those errors after the procedure has been completed. The idea is to stop the error before it is imprinted into the motor memory of the learner. Therefore, as the instructor places their hand on the learner's hands, redirecting them to the accurate motor skill, they prevent the learner from incorporating an incorrect movement into their motor memory [3].

Guided practice is critical to skill acquisition and mastery. Time should be provided for the student to practice the procedure repeatedly under the guidance of an instructor who will redirect and provide feedback when necessary. As the learner becomes more comfortable with the procedure, demonstrating increased skill competence, the instructor's involvement in the procedure should decrease until the learner is essentially performing it without assistance. Practice without guidance can precipitate errors and imprinting of inappropriate actions, which is dangerous to patients and a disservice to the learner. Immediate feedback, both positive and negative, is invaluable throughout the learning process. More specifically, effective feedback is performance-based, highlighting portions of the procedure that were done well and pointing out areas for improvement with specific tips on how to improve the skill attempted [1, 5]. There will be occasions when the learner fails to successfully perform the entire procedure. It is important to create a positive learning experience in this scenario. One effective way to educate the learner regarding mistakes is a face-to-face debriefing session. It is most beneficial if this discussion takes place immediately after the procedure. In most cases, the learner will have a high level of self-awareness and be able to identify areas for improvement. Feedback by the instructor should be given in a positive way, first emphasizing the correct steps performed, then providing a constructive critique of any errors in technique, and finally encouraging the learner to reattempt the procedure with guidance.

Once a basic procedure is mastered by a learner, the next step in skill acquisition is to present variations on that procedure. It is in this final step that learners may be introduced to the short-cuts or varied methods which instructors may use in their daily practice. They should be challenged to apply the procedure in difficult situations and learn alternative techniques to accomplish the desired outcome [5].

## Putting theory into practice

In reality, many physicians-in-training are still learning procedures within the framework of the "see one, do one, teach one" model. The transition to a more formalized, effective method for learning key procedural skills is difficult, as it requires more preparation on the part of both the learner and the teacher. In addition, the manpower hours required to teach and supervise learners practicing new procedures is considerable. There are various ways to implement the recommended teaching methods, including computer software models, low fidelity model practice, simulation labs, cadaver/animal labs, and bedside teaching on patients. Each of these teaching environments, when used within the framework of the teaching theories presented earlier in this chapter, can provide an opportunity for effective learning.

At the most basic level, simple teaching models are most effective when teaching the core motor activities required for a procedure. These models are often less expensive and more portable than simulators or cadavers, and they carry no risk of errors when compared with bedside teaching. As one study conducted by a surgery department demonstrates, using a simple model such as a pig thigh, to teach a surgical procedure led to significant improvements in overall performance by residents. The authors of this study noted that given the constraints of decreasing operating room time, and increased liability concerns for allowing junior residents to practice and learn on live patients, residents were not receiving adequate training in certain procedures. Therefore a brief training session was developed using the model of a pig thigh with a pre and post session evaluation. Residents demonstrated a significant increase in their post session scores, regardless of level of training or experience with the procedure in the past. The success of this basic teaching technique was primarily linked to the quality and the availability of immediate feedback for the learners as they practiced the procedure in the session. As noted by the authors, a simple tool, such as a pig thigh, provides an opportunity for new learners to practice a procedure in a safe, inexpensive environment with close mentoring prior to direct patient contact in the operating room [6].

A more costly, but increasingly popular tool for teaching multiple aspects of medicine, including procedural education, is the simulator model. Benefits of employing this model versus a human model include increased safety, the ability to practice the same procedure multiple times in a single session, and the option of exploring the consequences of errors without the risk of harm to a patient. Although cadavers may provide the best approximation of the tactile and visual cues of a human-based procedure, technologic advances in materials sciences and computer-based models have provided for a close approximation in many cases. In addition, the interactive capability of a simulator model allows the instructor to create increasingly challenging circumstances for the learner. For example, a new learner may experience mentored practice placing a central line in a perfectly still, sedated simulator model initially. As the learner becomes more proficient, the simulator may be mani-pulated to provide a patient with low blood volume and easily collapsible veins to present a realistic challenge to the learner, therefore encouraging advanced skill acquisition. As with any other teaching model, the key component which has shown to result in successful skill acquisition is guided, consistent practice with a decreasing role of the instructor in the actual performance of the procedure as the learner becomes more proficient [7].

Similarly, the cadaver lab provides an opportunity to learn and practice invasive procedures without posing any threat to a patient. The limitations of this modality include the availability of human cadavers and the expense involved. Use of human cadavers provides accurate human anatomy with all the natural variations. Palpation of landmarks and subtle anatomic differences provide a more realistic experience for the learner. At times, complications that cannot be recreated in a simulator model allow for a better education. An example includes inability to advance a guide wire in a cannulated vein, or the need for suctioning of an airway while teaching direct laryngoscopy. There are also disadvantages to the anatomic and pathologic differences among cadavers. For example, venous thromboses can prevent flash back in central line access attempts and pleural adhesions can complicate placement of chest tubes. These variations can result in inconsistent learning among a cohort of students. Finally, the safety of all participants must be ensured by screening donors for communicable infections.

All of the aforementioned settings are effective precursors to bedside procedural learning. As the optimal setting for the advanced learner, bedside teaching provides the opportunity for one-on-one instruction with a master in the procedure on a real live patient. Although performance of the procedure can be guided by the expert, it is preferable when the learner feels comfortable with the basic steps of the procedure and has performed it in other settings prior to performing it at the bedside. Immediate feedback can be provided by both the educator and the patient. Although performing a procedure at the bedside should be reserved for those learners who have already been instructed regarding the procedure and practiced it in a more structured setting, other phases of procedural learning can successfully occur at the bedside. For example, a medical student who has only read about a procedure can accomplish the visualization phase of learning at the bedside by observing the teacher performing the procedure in a fluid manner from start to finish. Those who have observed the procedure once or twice can be asked to verbalize the procedure and prompt the expert performing the procedure regarding the next step to be taken and how it is to be done. In addition, the learner who has attempted a procedure in lab previously can be guided to assist in performance of certain steps of the procedure, whereas the overall performance is primarily by the teacher. As the learner builds experience at the bedside, the number of steps which they perform can be increased until they are able to attempt the entire procedure under direct guidance. In this manner, the bedside can be a suitable environment for a variety of levels of learning procedural skills. The key is to recognize the stage of the learner and create the appropriate, safe experience based on that stage of learning.

## Creating a procedural education elective for preclinical medical students

Many educators and clinicians have commented that medical school is the optimal time in physician training to teach basic procedural skills. As medical students have less direct patient care responsibilities, and more time to spend practicing acquired skills, many emergency medicine clerkships have designated space within their curricula for procedural education. Beyond the basic skills learned at the bedside, specific procedural skills sessions using cadavers and simulators are now an increasingly popular way to provide exposure to clinical procedures for these new learners within a safe, well-supervised environment. Even outside of the framework of a rotation in emergency medicine, many medical schools employ the skills of emergency physicians when planning preclinical procedural education sessions for rising second and third year medical students.

One inventive approach to this has been demonstrated at Stanford University in the form of a very popular preclinical elective known as Essential Procedures in Emergency Medicine (EPEM). The structure of this course is modeled on the principles of motor-based learning presented in this chapter. In summary, educational sessions of 2 hours duration twice weekly throughout a quarter expose these students to procedural education prior to their clinical rotations. For each procedure there is a pre-session reading assignment, an interactive didactic session, followed by a demonstration of the procedure by an instructor, and then guided practice of the procedure. Furthermore, each student spends a set number of hours in the ED under the guidance of physicians and nurses performing procedures on live patients. Finally, there is a cadaver lab session in which more invasive and rare procedures, such as cricothyroidotomy, tube thoracostomy, and central venous access, are practiced with expert assistance and supervision [8].

Student evaluation includes a written examination regarding the basic indications, materials, contraindications, and steps for a given procedure, as well as a practical examination in which the student performs certain procedures in front of an instructor while responding to questions regarding that procedure. To evaluate the effectiveness of this course, EPEM students' performance in their clinical rotations was compared with their classmates who did not participate in this elective. The results demonstrated that EPEM students had significantly higher scores on procedural performance during their emergency medicine and internal medicine clinical rotations. In addition, enrollment in the elective exceeded expectations during the years studied, demonstrating that preclinical medical students are very interested in having this type of experience prior to their clinical rotations. Overall, this course presents a successful example of procedural education for early learners that takes into account the educational theory of motor skills acquisition and uses multiple models for guided practice and learning with feedback. It provides a venue for students to learn basic procedures in a prescribed sequence from master teachers, rather than in the unstructured and often inexperienced hands of residents during their clinical rotations [8].

---

## Summary point

Teaching procedures is essential to the practice of academic emergency medicine. When based on the principles of psychomotor learning (Tables 5.2 and 5.3), procedural teaching can be both enjoyable and successful for all parties involved.

**Table 5.2** Key points in procedural Education.

---

- Be sure the learner understands the basis for the procedure.
- Have the learner observe the procedure (text book, video, live).
- Break down the procedure into small digestible components.
- Ask the trainee to verbally describe each aspect of the procedure.
- Inform the patient that a student will be involved in the procedure and that you will be giving direction and supervising.
- Tell the learner to expect to have an error corrected immediately by redirecting their hand or stopping and starting fresh.
- Provide regular opportunities for guided practice.

---

**Table 5.3** Common pitfalls to avoid.

---

- Taking the micro skills required to perform a complex procedure for granted.
- Inadequate selection and preparation of an appropriate learning environment.
- Demonstrating a procedure with the observer positioned in a different orientation than that which the procedure is performed.
- Teaching inconsistent, varied versions of the same procedure.
- Failure to immediately correct an error during a procedure.

# References

1. The University of Kansas School of Medicine – Wichita. Teaching Clinical Skills [document on the Internet]. The University of Kansas School of Medicine – Wichita; [cited September 21, 2007]. Available from: http://wichita.kumc.edu/preceptor/teachingClinicalSkills2.html
2. George JH, Doto FX. A simple five-step method for teaching clinical skills. *Fam Med* 2001; 33(8): 577–578.
3. Gallery ME. Teaching clinical skills. In: Whiteside MF, Geist MA, eds. *The Emergency Medicine Teaching Fellowship Manual.* ACEP, 2001. module 2.3.1–11 *ACEP teaching fellowship manual,* Dallas, Texas.
4. Wang TS, Schwartz JL, Karimipour DJ, Orringer JS, Hamilton T, Johnson TM. An education theory-based method to teach a procedural skill. *Arch Dermatol* 2004; 140: 1357–1361.
5. McLeod PJ, Steinert Y, Trudel J, Gottesman R. Seven principles for teaching procedural and technical skills. *Acad Med* 2001; 76(10): 1080.
6. Wanzel KR, Matsumoto ED, Hamstra SJ, Anastakis DJ. Teaching technical skills: training on a simple, inexpensive and portable model. *J Am Soc Plast Reconstr Surg* 2002; 109(1): 258–264.
7. Kneebone R. Evaluating clinical simulations for learning procedural skills: a theory-based approach. *Acad Med* 2005; 80(6): 549–553.
8. Van der Vlugt TM, Harter PM. Teaching procedural skills to medical students: one institution's experience with an emergency procedures course. *Ann Emerg Med* 2002; 40(1): 41–49.

## CHAPTER 6

# Providing feedback in the emergency department

*David A. Wald[1], Esther K. Choo[2]*
[1]*Department of Emergency Medicine, Temple University School of Medicine, Wynnewood, PA, USA*
[2]*Research Fellow & Clinical Instructor, Department of Emergency Medicine, Oregon Health & Science University, Portland, OR, USA*

## Introduction

Feedback is an essential part of the medical education process. In the right hands, it can be a persuasive teaching tool that shapes the attitudes and behaviors of learners. By definition, feedback in the setting of clinical medical education refers to information describing a learner's performance in a specific activity with the goal of guiding their future performance in that same or other related activity [1]. Feedback can be viewed as "descriptive information" given to the learner by an unbiased observer. Keeping this in mind, the primary goal of giving feedback should be to provide the learner with an objective assessment of his or her performance. By providing feedback, the teacher can reinforce a job well done, alert the learner about an area of weakness, and provide some direction or recommendation on how to improve or remediate clinical performance [2]. Without feedback, mistakes go uncorrected and good performance is not reinforced. In essence, feedback is analogous to performance improvement. Educational feedback is intended to stimulate a behavioral change in the learner.

As teachers, we have a professional and ethical obligation to our learners. One can think of the relationship that a teacher has with a learner as analogous to that of a coach and an athlete. A coach, especially one of elite athletes, is a professional at improving performance through feedback. As mentors to medical students and physicians in training we effectively serve as educational coaches.

*Practical Teaching in Emergency Medicine,* 1st edition. Edited by R Rogers, A Mattu, M Winters & J Martinez. ©2009 Blackwell Publishing, ISBN: 9781405176224

A successful coach will alter his or her feedback style to the individual needs of the athlete or learner, at times supportive, at times cajoling, and if necessary, at times reprimanding [3].

In an ideal learning environment, trainees would have greater continuity with their preceptors and there would be ample opportunity for direct observation of a learner's clinical and procedural skills. This is, however, not the case in the emergency department (ED), where a variety of factors including: constant interruptions, endless unexpected events, high acuity case mix, and shift work scheduling limits the time available for clinical teaching. Obstacles to teaching in the ED are reviewed in greater detail in a different chapter of this text. Because of these barriers, faculty and senior emergency medicine (EM) trainees need to adapt their feedback delivery techniques both to the individual learner and to the specific clinical scenario at hand.

## General guidelines for providing effective feedback

Despite the many obstacles to teaching, feedback can be readily incorporated as an effective teaching tool into the unique educational environment of the ED. The classic paper by Ende delineates many of the principles of providing effective feedback in the clinical setting [1]. These techniques and others will be reviewed in this chapter with an emphasis on approaches that work well in the ED (Table 6.1). As an aside, the preceptor should have a heightened awareness of the effect of providing feedback in front of a patient. Each of us has our own idiosyncrasies and opinions with regards to certain clinical skills. It is important to pass this knowledge on to our learners in a way that respects their autonomy without undermining the confidence that the patient has in their ability. An example that I can recall from my own residency training (David A. Wald) involved the repair of a laceration on a young child's forehead. The attending physician entered the examination room as I was about to begin the procedure. He recommended that I approach the laceration in a particular fashion. I viewed his recommendations as guidance and feedback on how I should approach the laceration. However, the patient's father viewed this as a reflection of my inexperience and proceeded to question if I was confident in my ability to repair the laceration. Similar educational or feedback goals could be met without detracting from the autonomy of the trainee; a better way to handle this and similar cases would be to discuss certain

**Table 6.1** Ten guidelines for effective feedback in the ED.

| | |
|---|---|
| I | Provide positive feedback |
| II | Make observations of specific behaviors or actions |
| III | Provide constructive feedback |
| IV | Elicit learner self-assessment |
| V | Be well timed |
| VI | Focus on areas that the learner can control or modify |
| VII | Use language that is nonjudgmental and non-evaluative |
| VIII | Make feedback a joint venture |
| IX | Incorporate feedback into teaching models |
| X | Assist in developing strategies for improvement |

aspects of the procedure away from the presence of the patient or family, or to guide the trainee at the bedside using non-verbal cues.

When providing feedback we recommend keeping the following in mind.

## I Provide positive feedback

Instructors should provide positive feedback, praising the learner for a job well done. This is not to say that feedback should be laced with commonly used descriptors such as "good job" or "you worked hard today." Although there is a time and place for comments such as these – certainly after a tough case or at the end of a busy shift – they offer little in the way of substance, and are likely to be quickly discarded by the learner. It is more helpful to end a shift with specific praise, something to the effect of, "You did a really good job today. When we were talking about Ms. Jones earlier, you presented her case in a clear and organized fashion and came up with a focused assessment and management plan. I also liked the way that you explained the diagnosis to her and answered her questions." This additional information can emphasize exactly what the learner did well, reinforcing attitudes and behaviors that are favorable. Keep in mind that positive reinforcement is always beneficial; however, if linked to specific behaviors, the feedback may have longer lasting effects.

## II Make observations of specific behaviors or actions

A key to providing meaningful feedback is to focus on specific behaviors or actions and not focus on issues that are unlikely to be modified such as certain personality traits. Remember, the focus should generally be on what the learner does or does not do as opposed to the learner themselves. This can best be accomplished by having the specific feedback be based on direct observation of clinical performance. Direct observation allows the teacher an opportunity to best assess specific core competencies such as interpersonal and communication skills. It is also important to be descriptive and specific. For example, if a student generated a poor differential diagnosis for one of his or her patients with right upper quadrant abdominal pain, feedback can be provided by simply saying; "In addition to the causes of right upper quadrant pain that you mentioned, I would also consider cholelithiasis and cholecystitis."

## III  Provide constructive feedback

Feedback should serve to provide direction as to how a learner can improve his or her clinical performance [4]. Constructive feedback can prevent certain actions or behaviors from being incorporated into the learner's routine. Although all feedback should be descriptive and specific, this is particularly important when providing feedback that may be perceived as negative by the learner. As a result of the inherent difficulty in initiating a conversation about "negative" aspects of performance, some teachers may avoid being direct and forthright with the learner. When "negative" or constructive feedback is necessary, an approach that is often recommended is to initiate the session with positive comments, followed by constructive criticism, and conclude with additional positive comments: the so called "feedback sandwich." Feedback using this type of approach is more palatable, both for the instructor to deliver and for the learner to receive. Remember, providing or receiving negative feedback often creates anxiety for both the teacher and the learner. Because of this, an emphasis should be made on providing constructive feedback with the goal of correcting observed deficiencies in order to shape future behavior.

## IV  Elicit self-assessment

One approach to consider when conducting a feedback session is to elicit learner self-assessment [5]. This allows the learner to initiate the conversation by expressing their view of their own performance. This "self-assessment" technique usually raises many of the same issues that the teacher wanted to make, but allows the learner to feel more psychologically invested in the process. At times, this approach may bring up other concerns that are equally important to the learner. Self-assessment sessions can often be initiated by the teacher posing various open ended questions to the learner;

"How do you feel that you performed today?," "Is there anything that you think you could have done better today?," "Is there anything that you feel you need to work on?"

Self-assessment is fundamental to the concept of self-directed learning and the maintenance of professional competence [6]. A key aspect of learner self-assessment is the assumption that a learner can accurately self-assess his or her clinical performance. As a teacher, we must keep in mind that the ability to accurately self-assess ones own clinical performance may not always be a given. In fact, some learners with the greatest deficiencies (those least competent) may have poor insight into their own clinical performance [7]. Because of this, self-assessment should not be provided in isolation, but should be coupled with feedback based on direct observation of clinical domains. The lack of self-awareness of a learner regarding clinical competence or perhaps incompetence is one of the greatest teacher – learner challenges.

## V Be well timed

Timing of feedback is critical. To be most effective, it should be given immediately, as the window of opportunity to comment on a particular behavior or action is relatively narrow. It makes intuitive sense that feedback should be provided when the event is still fresh in the mind of both the learner and the teacher. This is applicable to any number of clinical scenarios, from patient interviewing to physical examination, to procedural skills. Suppose you observe a learner examining a patient with suspected pneumonia. Afterwards, you might tell him, "I noticed that you only listened to the anterior lung fields when you examined the patient. You should listen to both anterior and posterior lung fields, especially when evaluating a patient with cardiopulmonary symptoms." Since the exam just happened, it would be easier for the learner to recall that he did not listen to the posterior lung fields and resolve to alter this behavior with future patient encounters. Constructive criticism of a brief, almost trivial observation such as this may have lasting effects on the learner if provided on the spot shortly after the observed behavior, especially if the feedback is presented in a constructive manner.

## VI Focus on areas that the learner can control and modify

Feedback in the ED is often delivered in brief, informal sessions, focusing on issues that the learner has the power to change, modify or improve within the confines of the rotation, such as a discrete clinical skill or knowledge deficit. Brief feedback can occur at the bedside while observing a learner perform a clinical or procedural skill, or away from the bedside at the conclusion of a patient encounter. Try to provide information in easily digestible portions, rather than inundating the learner with multifaceted feedback. This approach is realistic in a clinical setting in which many of the teachable moments are unplanned and unscripted and time is in short supply. As we are all well aware of, trying to modify certain personality traits of learners is often fraught with frustration on both the part of the teacher and learner. The key point is that feedback should be behaviorally anchored. We all know that limited time is available in a busy ED for direct observation. Because of this, at times we are left with providing feedback on case presentation skills and indirectly the history and physical examination. It will be logistically easier, often because of time constraints, to provide feedback on the "product" of the patient interview as opposed to the interview itself, the "process," although each is equally important.

## VII Language should be nonjudgmental and non-evaluative

As a teacher, communication skills are as important when providing feedback to a learner as they are in talking to patients and professional colleagues. Specifically, language should be nonjudgmental and should convey respect for the learner as an individual. The instructor should not attempt to evaluate the learner's personal qualities or overall level of skill or ability, but confine comments to the situation at hand and observable actions or behaviors.

Take for example, a case in which a junior trainee commits a common diagnostic error, premature closure. The patient is a 34-year-old female who presents with calf pain and swelling five days after a motor vehicle accident (MVA). The trainee latches on to the diagnosis of muscle strain and does not entertain the possibility that the patient could have developed a deep venous thrombosis (DVT). The skilled teacher would approach feedback in this case in a way that is both constructive and conducive to learning, avoiding humiliation or discouragement. Using such an approach, you might state to the learner; "I can see your point. Ms. Smith was involved in an MVA 5 days ago and presents with a tender and swollen right calf. Her complaints may very well be the result of musculoskeletal trauma to her leg, but I believe that we should consider DVT as a possible explanation for her complaint, as this would be a very important diagnosis not to miss." This allows the preceptor to acknowledge the trainee's assessment of the case yet redirect with a suggestive style of teaching that is not offensive, placing emphasis on the clinically important points of the case rather than the learner's deficiency.

## VIII  Make feedback a joint venture

An important concept to convey to the learner is that feedback is a joint venture. The principle shareholder, the learner, should take charge by soliciting feedback from their preceptors if they feel that they are not receiving adequate feedback. A feedback discrepancy has been noted in a study by Gil *et al.* [8], in which the authors identified substantial differences between the amount of feedback faculty perceived providing from that which medical students perceived receiving. Instructors may need to be explicit whenever there is concern that the learner is not receptive to or aware of receiving feedback. This may be accomplished by beginning a discussion with a student or trainee by stating, "I'd like to provide you with some feedback on your performance." It may require specifically stating that feedback is about to be given for the learner to realize this.

## IX  Incorporate feedback into teaching models

Feedback does not have to be provided in isolation. Frequently feedback is incorporated into various teaching models. One such model, the One Minute Clinical Preceptor [9], consists of five "microskills" that have been shown to be effective: (1) get a commitment from the learner, (2) probe the learner for their underlying reasoning, (3) teach general rules, (4) provide positive feedback, and (5) correct errors. Feedback is just one facet of a much broader continuum of medical education that usually starts by creating a comfortable, friendly learning environment.

Imagine a clinical scenario in which you as the supervising physician are observing a trainee perform an incision and drainage of a cutaneous abscess. As the learner proceeds through each step of the procedure – patient consent, equipment preparation, skin preparation, infiltration of local anesthesia, and so on – you might ask about the reasoning behind individual actions, offer guidance or suggestions about specific skills, comment positively on things done well, and correct any errors. Simply interacting with the learner in this informal, natural way, you have utilized an effective model for feedback delivery. One study involving medical students has shown that trainees indeed receive more instructional feedback if selected procedural skills are directly observed [10]. To be most effective, feedback should be explicitly linked to direct observation of certain actions or behaviors.

## X Assist in developing strategies for improvement

Constructive feedback should be followed by an action plan for improving performance. On a number of levels, this may be one of the most important aspects of the feedback process. In our role as teachers, we are charged with the responsibility of guiding our learners through the educational process. Because of this, it is necessary to provide the learners with direction on how they may improve their clinical performance. We should be ready to offer resources, ideas, or time, in order to help a learner address any noted deficiencies. This may be as simple as having the learner repeat the procedural skill while incorporating the instructor's suggestions, assigning a book chapter or review article to read, or spending time reviewing cases, ECG's or radiographs. Real time suggestions for improving clinical performance may also be provided during brief direct observation sessions. Some learners will be capable of creating an individualized educational plan, but most if not all will benefit from the teacher who will be available to monitor progress and assist in both articulating and implementing the plan.

## Additional feedback methods and tools

### Feedback cards

A number of authors have reported on a simplified method for providing effective feedback to learners [11–13]. These reports all revolve around using some sort of feedback card, completed by the preceptor to ensure that feedback occurs and to enhance the quantity and quality of feedback. The authors have had success using a modified feedback note card developed at the Medical College of Wisconsin [11]. A feedback note system such as this can easily be incorporated into the daily shift evaluation process that many EM clerkships use. However, faculty and resident educational development sessions and administrative buy-in are critical to ensuring the consistency and success of such a program.

### Written feedback/evaluation

In the busy ED, time and patient related constraints might prevent us from adequately reflecting on a trainee's performance. Because of this, it is sometimes necessary to follow up on an interaction with a learner with written comments. This may be accomplished by completing an end of rotation written evaluation form or in a follow-up email that can allow the teacher to provide an extended reflection on the trainee's performance, hopefully supplementing the bedside feedback already provided.

Faculty are frequently called upon to complete daily shift evaluations or end-of-rotation evaluations of learners. A clerkship or rotation grade may then be determined based on a composite of these evaluations. Too often, preceptors do not make full use of this opportunity to deliver feedback. Written communication gives us the advantage of being more calculating in our assessment and limiting any potential disconnect between the perceived intent and the likely perception of comments. Written comments should routinely support prior feedback and not surprise the learner with unfavorable comments that have been withheld throughout the rotation due to the tendency to avoid giving negative feedback.

In general, the same guidelines proposed for verbal feedback should be adhered to when providing written feedback. A clerkship evaluation form is an appropriate venue to provide constructive comments so that learners can modify behavior or actions as needed or to provide praise for a job well done. Comments should be as specific as possible and should include recommendations for performance improvement.

**Formal feedback sessions**

A more formal approach to providing feedback can occur in the ED at the conclusion of a clinical shift [14]. For this type of feedback session to have the greatest impact on the learner, it should be uninterrupted whenever possible. Formal feedback can still be brief, but is provided away from the bedside in a more quiet and controlled area. These sessions in general are more interactive than "brief" sessions, should allow learners a chance for questions and rebuttal, and should be goal oriented, with specific topics on the instructor's agenda. These type of sessions can even occur prior to the start of a clinical rotation and may be an ideal time to review the learning objectives of the rotation and to better understand the individual learner's goals that they may have for their own performance. This type of meeting can essentially set the tone for future feedback sessions.

Trainees who require more extensive feedback due to documented unprofessional behavior or a trend of less-than-expected clinical performance may benefit from "major" feedback sessions of 15 to 30 minutes. Major feedback sessions can be scheduled at the midpoint or end of a clinical rotation and are best held outside of the patient care setting in the instructor's office. Semiannual feedback sessions commonly provided to EM trainees throughout their education may also be used to address major deficiencies or concerns.

### Feedback and the accreditation process

The process of providing formal feedback for trainees is integral to both the undergraduate and graduate medical education accreditation process. The U.S. Department of Education recognizes the Liaison Committee on Medical Education (LCME) for the accreditation of medical education programs leading to the M.D. degree in the U.S. For Canadian medical education programs, the LCME engages in accreditation in collaboration with the Committee on Accreditation of Canadian Medical Schools (CACMS). The LCME outlines this expectation in the most recent version (June, 2006) of the standards for accreditation of medical education programs [15]. The standards mandate that the directors of all courses and clerkships design and implement a system of formative and summative evaluation of student achievement. It is further expected that courses and clerkships provide students with formal feedback during the experience so that they may understand and remediate their deficiencies. In addition, EM residency training programs in the U.S. should provide each resident with semiannual evaluations of performance with feedback. This expectation is described in the common program requirements (effective July, 2007) set forth by the Accreditation Council for Graduate Medical Education (ACGME), the governing body responsible for accrediting U.S. graduate medical education training programs [16].

### Faculty/trainee development

Like any other skill, feedback requires training and practice. However well-intentioned individual instructors are, feedback is unlikely to occur on a meaningful level in the ED without a substantial amount of administrative support and resources dedicated to the education of faculty and senior trainees. There is no shortage of materials for training instructors, as well as materials specifically designed for teaching and feedback delivery in the fast-paced environment of the ED [17–19]. Feedback training can occur via faculty development programs that include feedback coaching as part of the curriculum (e.g., the Stanford Faculty Development Program) or through other departmental or medical school supported faculty development courses. Trainees may benefit from a proposed "Resident-As-Teacher" curriculum for EM, which includes a module on giving effective feedback [18].

### Feedback versus evaluation

An important distinction to be aware of is the difference between feedback and evaluation [20]. Feedback is a formative process that can occur on a day-to-day or even moment-to-moment basis. Evaluation provides a summary description of performance as it relates to the achievement of specific learning objectives and may be associated with rendering a clerkship or rotation grade. Although a distinction exists, there is at times an overlap between feedback and evaluation both in form and in intent. Both are important for the medical education process and the learner to move forward.

## Conclusion

Feedback is a crucial part of the training of medical students and trainees. Even in the busy ED environment, instructors can deliver effective feedback by using strategies outlined above and can easily incorporate the provision of feedback into other teachable moments. Individual instructors have the option of a variety of methods of feedback delivery to enhance the learning and guide the future performance of both students and trainees.

---

### Summary points

Feedback in clinical medical education should be:
- Descriptive, based on specific observations
- An objective assessment of performance
- Intended to stimulate change in the behavior of the learner.

---

## References

1. Ende J. Feedback in Clinical Medical Education. *JAMA* 1983; 250: 777–781.
2. Lucas JH, Stallworth JR. Providing difficult feedback: TIPS for the problem learner. *Fam Med* 2003; 35(8): 544–546.

3. Sheehan JT. Feedback: Giving and Receiving. *J Med Educ* 1984; 59: 913.

4. Hewson M, Little M. Giving Feedback in Medical Education: Verification of Recommended Techniques. *J Gen Intern Med* 1998; 13: 111–116.

5. Branch W, Paranjabe A. Feedback and Reflection: Teaching Methods for Clinical Settings. *Acad Med* 2002; 77: 1185–1188.

6. Ward M, Gruppen L, Regehr G. Measuring Self-Assessment: Current State of the Art. *Advance Health Sci Educ* 2002; 7: 63–80.

7. Hodges B, Regehr G, Martin D. Difficulty in Recognizing One's Own Incompetence: Novice Physicians Who Are Unskilled and Unaware of it. *Acad Med* 2001; 76: s87–s89.

8. Gil D, Heins M, Jones P. Perceptions of Medical School Faculty Members and Students on Clinical Clerkship Feedback. *J Med Educ* 1984; 59: 856–864.

9. Furney S, Orsini A, Orsetti K, *et al.* The One Minute Clinical Preceptor. *J Gen Intern Med* 2001; 16(9): 620–624.

10. Wald DA, Barrett J. Procedural Observation of Medical Students: Is There a Relationship between Direct Observation and Procedural Instruction and Assistance? *Acad Emerg Med* 2004; 11: 500.

11. Schum T, Krippendorf R. Feedback Notes: A System for Feedback to Students and Residents. Advanced Education Faculty Development Group. *Acad Med* 2000; 75(5): 556–557.

12. Prystowsky J, DaRosa D. A Learning Prescription Permits Feedback on Feedback. *Am J Surg* 2003; 185: 264–267.

13. Paukert J, Richards M, Olney C. An Encounter Card System for Increasing Feedback to Students. *Am J Surg* 2002; 183: 300–304.

14. Manthey D, Coates W, Ander D. Report of the Task Force on National Fourth Year Medical Student Emergency Medicine Curriculum Guide. *Ann Emerg Med* 2005; 47: e1–e7.

15. Functions and Structure of a Medical School. *Liaison Committee on Medical Education*. Updated June 2006. Available at: http://www.lcme.org/functions2006june.pdf.

16. Common Program Requirements. Available at: http://www.acgme.org/acWebsite/dutyHours/dh_dutyhoursCommonPR07012007.pdf.

17. Richardson B. Feedback. *Acad Emerg Med* 2004; 11(12): e1281–e1285.

18. Farrell SE, Pacella C, Egan D, *et al.* Resident-as-teacher: A suggested curriculum for emergency medicine. *Acad Emerg Med* 2006; 13(6): 677–679.

19. Henderson P, Ferguson-Smith AC, Johnson MH. Developing essential professional skills: A framework for teaching and learning about feedback. *BMC Med Educ* 2005; 5(1): 11.

20. Quattlebaum T. Techniques for evaluating residents and residency programs. *Pediatrics* 1996; 98(6 Pt 2): 1277–1283.

# CHAPTER 7

# The computer as a teaching tool

*Joshua S. Broder*
*Duke University Division of Emergency Medicine, Duke University Medical Center, Durham, NC, USA*

Computers provide a powerful tool for practical teaching in the emergency department (ED). The ability to access remote information means that no ED – from the busiest county hospital to the quietest rural site – should be an educational backwater. Internet resources can be used to provide "virtual expertise" on the latest breakthroughs and the rarest conditions, allowing learners to benefit from the insights of distant gurus. Educators can use internet resources to illustrate a teaching point, to provide a skill-building exercise for the learner, or to enhance their own knowledge of a less familiar topic. For teaching programs with multiple clinical sites and variable day–night clinical schedules, computer-based learning can provide a consistent curriculum for students separated in both time and space. Internet-based resources can be tailored easily to the student's existing level of knowledge, and the sequence of information presented can be individualized, sometimes to a greater extent than in group classroom exercises. In the busiest clinical moments, computer-based teaching can keep the student productively occupied while the physician educator attends to patient care, with debriefing occurring at a later time.

Using online resources to augment student education is a pragmatic way of introducing students to both skills and content format that will likely remain with them for the rest of their careers. Between 1998 and 2003, available internet-based continuing medical education (CME) increased by 700% compared with 38% in

*Practical Teaching in Emergency Medicine,* 1st edition. Edited by R Rogers, A Mattu, M Winters & J Martinez. ©2009 Blackwell Publishing, ISBN: 9781405176224

total CME activities. At the same time, the number of physicians receiving CME credit for internet activities increased by 1400%, compared with a 64% increase for all CME [1, 2]. By 2006, a variety of internet activities accounted for 17,704 separate CME activities sponsored by the ACCME (Accreditation Council for Continuing Medical Education), accounting for 25% of total CME activities directly sponsored by the ACCME [3].

Are computers an effective means of delivering educational content? A number of studies have attempted to ferret out the educational impact of computer-based learning, compared with more traditional live lecture formats. Measures such as exam performance and satisfaction surveys suggest that well-implemented computer learning can match or outperform live classroom exercises, although an important part of many of these programs is some form of interaction with a live educator, for example through a real-time threaded discussion forum [4–8].

In this chapter, we will introduce a variety of educational exercises which you can employ during your next shift. For each exercise, one or more internet sites are suggested to get you started, but the constant evolution of web content means newer and better resources may be available to you. Search engines such as Google provide a rapid means of locating new resources, but we hope you will appreciate the short, selected lists we have provided – a Google search of "ECG" returns over 11 million hits! In addition, the student and teacher alike must be keenly aware of the source and quality of information obtained from the internet. Inaccurate information on the internet may be the result of many factors including the qualifications of the authors, how recently the information was updated to reflect new research findings, and conflicts of interest in funding sources. A reliable source should name its authors, provide its publication date, disclose its funding source, and list references where applicable. Positive study results may be contraindicated by future research or effect sizes may be shown to be smaller than originally stated in 16% of cases [9]. One of the most important educational points you can make is teaching the student to find and use only the most reliable information.

Each of these exercises can be based on the student's real patient. In addition, it is often thought provoking to ask the student about a hypothetical change in the patient's scenario, such as pregnancy, an allergy, a new medication, or a co-morbid illness. These variations can transform a seemingly mundane case into a valuable educational experience. For each of these exercises, a face-to-face discussion and debriefing are important – the computer is a tool to enhance your efficiency and effectiveness, but you remain the teacher.

Section 1: Improving patient care by locating and implementing evidence-based clinical guidelines
*Question: "What is the evidence-based method of diagnosing and treating condition X?"*
Students may be unaware that evidence-based, consensus guidelines exist for many conditions. Open this discussion by asking the student how they would manage the diagnosis or treatment of the patient. Try to ascertain the student's existing knowledge about the condition. Some of the most effective teaching can come from coaxing the student into recognizing his or her own knowledge deficit or frank misconception, and then leading the student to find the best information on that topic. A great Website for this situation is the National Guideline Clearinghouse: www.guidelines.gov. In addition, the American College of Emergency Physicians publishes its clinical policies at http://www.acep.org/practres.aspx?id= 30060&coll=1&collid=74 (Google "ACEP clinical policies"). In addition, most medical search engines such as PubMed allow restriction of searches to practice guidelines using a "Limits" feature.

**Suggested Website**
National Guidelines Clearinghouse        www.guidelines.gov

Section 2: Performing an effective and efficient evidence-based medicine (EBM) literature search for clinically meaningful answers during a busy shift
*Question: "What is the quality of evidence for treatment of condition X with treatment Y, or for diagnosis of condition X with modality Y?"*
Key to the future success of our students as physicians is the ability to find evidence efficiently, and to evaluate it for methodological rigor and internal and external validity. This is not just the domain of journal club but can be a topic for clinical learning and application. Students need to understand how to perform a rapid and appropriately targeted search in the ED and to evaluate the applicability of the research findings to their patients. Although practice guidelines can be the source for many diagnostic and therapeutic

decisions, they may be outdated, biased by industry sponsorship, or may not exist for the condition in question. Some great exercises include teaching a student to use the "Limits" field of search engines such as PubMed, OVID, or less traditional engines such as Google Scholar (www.scholar.google.com). Other search engines include pre-filtered specialty databases such as Best Evidence Topics from the *British Medical Journal*, the *Cochrane Database*, *ACP Journal Club*, and *Emergency Medical Abstracts*. Studies comparing these search engines have demonstrated that they compare favorably with broader search engines in identifying clinically useful evidence [10].

Many exercises are possible using medical search engines. Ask the student to structure the clinical question using the Patients/Interventions/Comparisons/Outcomes (PICO) model [10]. This model is demonstrated at the Centre for Evidence-Based Medicine webpage under the heading, "Asking Focused Questions" (Google "CEBM PICO"). Demonstrate to the student that the search term "myocardial infarction aspirin" retrieves 4714 hits in PubMed, whereas limiting the same search to "human," "English," "Randomized Controlled Trial," "Adult" and adding the term "mortality" reduces the number of hits to 276. Adding the search term "emergency" reduces the number of retrieved studies to 11, a reasonable number for the practicing physician to peruse during clinical care in the ED. An important corollary to this is to demonstrate to the student that a restricted search strategy can miss important information. For example, the search listed above misses the sentinel ISIS-2 study [11] showing the mortality benefit of aspirin … because this study was not conducted in the ED setting. To demonstrate this point further, ask the student to perform the same search in multiple engines and compare the results. Another exercise to refine the student's search capability is to pick a target study, such as NEXUS or ISIS-2, and ask the student to perform a search to answer a related clinical question. A clinically useful search strategy should retrieve the target study, and it may be useful to the student to experiment with various search strategies to see which is most effective in finding the clinically relevant evidence. A guide to performing clinically relevant searches was published in *Annals of Emergency Medicine* in 2003 and demonstrates several useful searches which can be reproduced by the student in the ED [10].

The Centre for Health Evidence (http://www.cche.net/usersguides/main.asp) publishes the Users' Guides to the Medical Literature, originally published in *JAMA*. These articles are a useful reference for you and the student and are divided by important clinical categories such as diagnosis, therapy, surrogate endpoints, and clinical prediction rules. Consider using these to highlight an EBM point, such as pre-test probability or internal and external validity. The Centre for Evidence-Based Medicine also has an excellent array of EBM tools which can be rapidly used to demonstrate an educational point. For example, their explanation of likelihood ratios using a likelihood ratio nomogram is a valuable tool for helping the student to visualize the degree of clinical certainty gleaned from a test result (http://www.cebm.net/index.aspx?o=1043, or Google "CEBM likelihood ratio").

## Suggested Websites

| | |
|---|---|
| PubMed | www.pubmed.org |
| Google Scholar | www.scholar.google.com |
| Emergency Medical Abstracts | http://ccme.org |
| Centre for Health Evidence | www.cche.net |
| Cochrane Library | www.cochrane.org |
| Best Evidence Topics | www.bestbets.org |
| Centre for Evidence-based Medicine | www.cebm.net |

Section 3: Improving utilization and interpretation of diagnostic imaging
*Questions: "Does your patient need imaging? Why? What kind? What findings will you look for? What if the imaging is normal? What is the radiation risk to the patient?"*
Understanding the role of diagnostic imaging in emergency conditions is a vital skill for the emergency physician, and one which can be divided into several important stages:

**a** Risk stratifying patients to determine who needs imaging
**b** Selecting the diagnostic imaging test appropriate to the condition
**c** Understanding the radiation risk of diagnostic imaging, and revising the imaging plan appropriately depending on patient factors
**d** Understanding the findings of the condition on diagnostic imaging
**e** Knowing the limits of diagnostic imaging, enabling the physician to recognize when a false negative imaging test may have occurred.

First, ascertain which stages of this process the student already can comfortably perform, and then engage him or her with learning more about those stages which are unfamiliar. For example, the student may be aware of the NEXUS rule and may be able to determine whether a patient with blunt trauma requires cervical spine imaging. But the student may be unaware of the usual imaging tests and may intend to perform cervical CT when plain films are sufficient. In addition, the student may not be familiar with the systemic evaluation of cervical plain films, and may be unaware of the limited sensitivity of plain films for fracture. The student may not know when additional imaging is needed to rule out fracture or ligamentous injury, or when a cervical collar and follow-up are indicated.

For each of the stages listed above, online resources can be useful tools. Clinical decision rules such as NEXUS; the Canadian Rules for C-spine and Head CT; the Ottawa ankle, foot, and knee rules; the Pittsburgh knee rule; and rules for venous thromboembolic disease risk stratification such as Well's Criteria can be introduced. MDCALC (www.MDCALC.com or Google "MDCALC") provides a variety of clinical decision rules, some with online calculators. The National Center for Emergency Medicine Infomatics (NCEMI.org) also provides calculator versions of many of these rules. Teaching the student to use and document these rules in the medical record is both good EBM and good clinical practice for billing and medical decision making.

A number of Websites have useful information demonstrating abnormal pathology on imaging and structured interpretation of imaging tests. EMPACS.org and mypacs.net both offer free searchable archives with annotated radiologic images. Both sites allow users to create bookmarked lists of interesting cases, and to view these in "quiz" or "training" modes to hide answers. EMPACS.org allows users to read library guides to the interpretation of head, chest, and abdominal CT. LearningRadiology.com provides many useful imaging references, including a series tailored for novices, called "Recognizing..." which highlights important imaging findings. A useful way to incorporate this clinically is to refer the student to a guide to the abnormality in question, such as "Recognizing a pneumothorax," asking the student to review this while the patient is undergoing the imaging test. This provides the basis for your discussion of the patient's test when completed.

Radiation risks of imaging studies are discussed in a brief but accessible publication by the International Commission on Radiologic Protections, entitled "Radiation and your Patient: A Guide for Medical Practitioners" (http://www.icrp.org/educational_area.asp). In addition, this site provides a brief PowerPoint outlining the risks of radiation in pregnancy. Introduce these questions by asking the student, "what will you tell your patient about the risks of the imaging study you are recommending?"

A discussion of pre- and post-test probability and likelihood ratios is an important part of helping the student to understand how to incorporate the diagnostic imaging results, positive or negative, into the clinical plan. Ask the student, "What is your pretest probability of disease? What is the likelihood ratio positive and negative for our imaging test? What is our post-test probability?" Refer the student to the Centre for Evidence-Based Medicine Website discussion on these topics (Google "CEBM likelihood ratio") for a clear, one page illustration of these topics. Engage the student to use a search engine to find the LR's for the imaging study.

## Suggested Websites

| | |
|---|---|
| National Center for Emergency Medicine Infomatics | www.ncemi.org |
| EMPACS | www.empacs.org |
| MYPACS | www.mypacs.net |
| Learning Radiology | http://learningradiology.com |
| Radiation exposure calculator | http://www.safety.duke.edu/ Radsafety |
| International Commission on Radiological Protection | www.icrp.org/educational_ area.asp |
| MDCALC | www.MDCALC.com |

Section 4: Enhancing systematic electrocardiogram interpretation
*Question: "Interpret this ECG systematically. What are the ECG abnormalities expected in condition X?"*
ECG analysis is clearly a core skill in emergency medicine (EM). Comprehensive online resources exist which can be a springboard for discussions of ECG abnormalities. This topic is so broad that the student may be overwhelmed by the amount of material available. First assess the student's baseline knowledge by asking him or her to perform a routine analysis of the ECG. Identify areas of weakness – an inability to recall the normal QRS duration, for example. Then send the student to an online resource with a specific question in mind – what is the normal QRS duration? What

happens to the QRS complex in a patient with Wolf-Parkinson-White Syndrome? The Alan E. Lindsay ECG Learning Center has an outstanding online course in ECG analysis, from beginning to advanced topics complete with quizzes.

Alternatively, give the student an online ECG to analyze and then compare this to the actual patient's ECG. The ECG Wave-Maven site has an excellent tool for this purpose – it allows you the teacher to search the library by diagnosis, and the ECG can then be displayed to the student with the answer hidden.

**Suggested Websites**

| | |
|---|---|
| ECG Library | www.ecglibrary.com |
| Wikipedia "ECG" | en.wikipedia.org/wiki/Electrocardiogram |
| The Alan E. Lindsay ECG Learning Center | library.med.utah.edu/kw/ecg/ |
| ECG primer | www.anaesthetist.com/icu/organs/ heart/ecg |
| ECG Wave-Maven | ecg.bidmc.harvard.edu/maven/ mavenmain.asp |

Section 5: Enhancing understanding of drug toxicity, interactions, and treatment

*Questions: What is the toxin? What is the toxic dose? Is decontamination helpful? Is an antidote available? What are the toxic effects? Are drug levels useful? What disposition is appropriate?*

Drug effects, interactions, and toxicology are great areas to explore with a student using computers. These are topics with a wealth of information not easily remembered, and since the practicing physician will often need to rely on online resources, introducing the student to these teaches not only medical knowledge but also practice skills which will be invaluable. Areas for teaching include pill identification, antidotes and decontamination, toxic effects including ECG changes associated with ingestions, and recommendations for observation. A fun exercise is to provide the student with an "unknown" pill and to ask the student to identify the potential toxin using an online identification tool. One such tool is http:// www.drugs.com/pill_identification.html, an index with images of pills, searchable by drug name, imprint, shape, and color.

Another site which can be useful is www.qtdrugs.org, which maintains up-to-date lists of drugs categorized by their risk of QT prolongation and subsequent torsades de pointes. The National

Center for Emergency Medicine Infomatics also maintains a Website (NCEMI) with multiple clinical calculators including toxicity nomograms for acetaminophen and ibuprofen.

Drug safety in pregnancy is an important topic which can be explored using a variety of resources. Ask the student, "Would this drug be safe to use in a pregnant patient? How will you answer the patient's questions about risk and benefit?" Up-to-date and ClinPharm are subscription services available through many medical centers which provide information on pregnancy and lactation risk. In addition, www.safefetus.com provides a list of medications categorized by FDA Pregnancy Risk Category.

Toxicity and antidote information is available through Micro-Medex, a subscription service. In addition, http://toxnet.nlm.nih.gov lists industrial and household chemicals with toxicity and treatment information. The limits of research on toxicology topics can also be a useful topic to explore with the student. This is a good opportunity to have the student search for randomized controlled trials of toxicity and treatment – if only to discover the paucity of evidence.

### Suggested Websites

| | |
|---|---|
| Drugs.com | www.drugs.com |
| Qt prolongation | www.qtdrugs.org |
| Drugs in pregnancy | www.safefetus.com |
| ToxNet drugs and household products | toxnet.nlm.nih.gov |

Section 6: Introducing a systematic approach to describing skin lesions

*Question: "Describe the skin lesion using color, morphology, pattern, organization, and location"*

Skin lesions are a frequent complaint in the ED, and education on this topic is sparse in most training programs. Computer resources can help you to teach the student to characterize a skin lesion systematically to facilitate diagnosis. DermAtlas from Johns Hopkins is a free collaborative archive of dermatologic cases with tools to aid in differential diagnosis. Ask the student to characterize the lesion by color, morphology, pattern, organization, and body location. With the aid of the online resource, have the student prepare a differential diagnosis for the lesion. As an alternative exercise, describe to the student a dangerous skin lesion, such as palpable purpura, using the systematic approach described above. Refer the learner to the online resource to find matching examples of this type of lesion, and again ask for the differential diagnosis.

## Suggested Website
DermAtlas          dermatlas.med.jhmi.edu/derm

Section 7: Enhancing the neurological exam, as well as an understanding of the NIH stroke scale and indications/contraindications for tissue plasminogen activator (TPA) for stroke
*Questions: "What is the patient's NIH stroke scale? Does the patient have contraindications to TPA administration?"*
Acute stroke represents a time-sensitive severe condition where teaching in the ED may appear impractical. However, this is an ideal scenario for hypothetical discussion. Ask the student, "Does the patient meet criteria for TPA administration? What is the patient's NIH stroke scale, and how does this influence your decision? Are contraindications present? What risks would you discuss with the patient and family?" The Foundation for Education and Research in Neurologic Emergencies (www.ferne.org) posts the NIH stroke scale, indications and contraindications for TPA, and a discussion of risks on its Website, under the heading "Clinical Practice → NIH stroke scale." Have the student print out the scale and perform it on a patient with a neurological complaint, as practice for a true ischemic stroke. Ask the student to time him or herself to see how this would impact the 3 hours window. Have the student time the patient's transportation to and from CT scan. Role-play the risk discussion with the student.

## Suggested Websites
Foundation for Education and          www.FERNE.org
  Research in Neurological
  Emergencies – links to GCS, NIH
  stroke scale
NIH Stroke Scale Training Online     http://www.strokeassociation.
                                      org/presenter.jhtml?identifier
                                      =3023009

Section 8: Enhancing the student's utilization of scoring systems, calculators and decision rules to provide the basis and documentation for care

*Question: "How do we make a structured risk assessment for condition X?"*

Clinical decision rules and scoring systems are growing in importance in EM and are an important topic for education. The strengths and weaknesses of these scores can be highlighted to the student using online resources. In addition, the student can learn to incorporate these scores into the medical record as documentation of medical decision making (for billing, medical-legal, and medical communication purposes). MDCALC provides an array of online scores and calculators commonly used in EM practice. These include the PORT score, Well's criteria, and Glasgow Coma Score. As an example of the use of these calculators, ask the student his planned disposition of a patient with pneumonia, and then demonstrate the PORT score for that patient. Explain to the student the limits of the PORT score, and role-play a discussion with a consultant using the PORT score to bolster a decision for admission. Ask the student to write a note for the medical record explaining the patient's PORT score and the disposition decision.

Online calculators can also be used to ease the sometimes difficult task of determining a patient's medication dose. MDCALC includes a glomerular filtration rate calculator which is useful when dosing patients with renal impairment. In addition, the Google search bar acts as a calculator which performs automatic unit conversion – and conveniently displays the unit conversion to allow the user to double-check the result. As an example, type "30 lbs*50 mg/kg=" and Google replies: "(30 pounds)*50(mg/kg) = 680.388555 milligrams." Type "38.1C to F" and Google produces: "38.1 degrees Celsius = 100.58 degrees Fahrenheit."

## Suggested Websites

Google calculator          www.google.com
MDcalc                     www.mdcalc.com

Section 9: Improving the student's understanding of normal changes in pregnancy, pregnancy complications, radiation risks in pregnancy, and contraindications of medications in pregnancy

*Questions: "What are some expected lab and vital sign changes in pregnancy? What classes of drugs are safe in pregnancy? What is the risk of imaging in pregnancy?"*

The pregnant patient in the ED presents a common scenario for education on drug and radiation risks, complications of pregnancy, and normal physiological changes. We have discussed above some online resources for drug and radiation information to share with the student. Another common theme is the correlation between human chorionic gonadotropin (HCG) measurements and normal fetal development. Explore with the student the range of expected HCG values in a patient, based on last menstrual period date. Ask the student to predict the HCG value in 48 hours, assuming the pregnancy is normal. Ask the student to consider the expected ultrasound findings at a given HCG level, assuming a normal pregnancy – and to explain the concept of the discriminatory zone. Change the scenario to a possible ectopic pregnancy and ask the student to reflect on the possible HCG values. Emedicine provides clear explanations of these topics, as well as many other EM subjects. Perinatology (www.perinatology.com) provides links to a variety of specialty topics and calculators relevant to the pregnant women and fetus.

### Suggested Websites
| | |
|---|---|
| CDC | http://www.bt.cdc.gov/radiation/prenatal.asp |
| Perinatology | http://www.perinatology.com/exposures/ |
| | Physical/Xray.htm |
| Emedicine | www.emedicine.com |

Section 10: Reinforcing the importance of clear communication and use of fluent translators for non-English speaking patients
*Question: "Does your patient speak fluent English? Do you speak your patient's primary language fluently? Could your patient have misunderstood your questions or instructions?"*
Non-English speakers are an important segment of the ED patient population, and miscommunication can impair diagnosis, as well as compliance with treatment plan and follow-up. Interpreters are underutilized [12] in the ED, and students with moderate language ability may be tempted to rely on their own interpretation or that of a family member, rather than engaging a professional interpreter. An exercise to emphasize the need for interpreter services is to have the student write discharge instructions using a web-based translation program, such as translate.google.com or Yahoo's Babelfish. Have the student translate the instructions from English to the target language and then back to English. If the resulting English instructions differ substantially from the original instructions, it is likely that the translation was confusing or imprecise. Ask your live interpreter to review the instructions with the

student for mistranslations. This may reinforce for the student the possibility that they may have misconstrued the patient's meaning of a word during the interview, or that their discharge instructions could be erroneous. Although computer translation programs are improving, errors in translation remain a potential threat.

### Suggested Websites

| | |
|---|---|
| Google translator | translate.google.com |
| AltaVista Babelfish | babelfish.altavista.com |

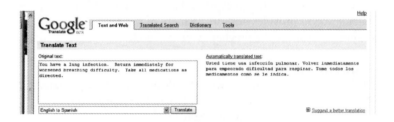

## Top 10 recommended Websites to use during a shift

| Topics | Web address* |
|---|---|
| Guidelines in emergency medicine | guidelines.gov |
| Evidence-based medicine literature searches | cche.net |
| Medical images | unmc.edu/library/reference/medimage.html |
| ECG interpretation | library.med.utah.edu/kw/ecg |
| Drugs and toxicology | drugs.com |
| Dermatology | dermatlas.med.jhmi.edu |
| Neurology | ferne.org |
| Clinical Decision Rules and Scores | mdcalc.com |
| Pregnancy | perinatology.com |
| Translation | translate.google.com |

*Shortest web address for Internet Explorer and Firefox provided. User may be redirected to a different address.

## Summary

Online computer resources provide outstanding tools to facilitate education in the ED. They allow sharing of medical knowledge, exploration of concepts in clinical thinking such as pre-test probability, and interpretation of clinical data such as ECGs and imaging studies. The role of the educator remains paramount, and framing the relevant question and debriefing the student are vital to ensure that the student learns and retains the information and skills essential to emergency medical care.

---

### Summary points

1. Computers are an effective tool for teaching content and clinically useful skills
2. The role of the educator remains paramount – debriefing is essential
3. Computer-based exercises can assist students to:
   - improve patient care by locating and implementing evidence-based clinical guidelines
   - perform an effective and efficient EBM literature search for clinically meaningful answers
   - improve utilization, and interpretation of diagnostic imaging
   - practice systematic ECG interpretation
   - understand drug toxicity, interactions, and treatment
   - describe skin lesions systematically
   - perform a thorough neurological exam
   - apply the NIH stroke scale
   - recognize indications/contraindications for TPA for stroke
   - utilize scoring systems, calculators, and clinical decision rules to provide the basis and documentation for care
   - understand normal changes in pregnancy, pregnancy complications, radiation risks in pregnancy, and contraindications of medications in pregnancy
   - reinforce clear communication and use of fluent translators for non-English speaking patients.

---

## References

1. Education ACfCM. Accreditation Council for Continuing Medical Education. ACCME Annual Report Data 2003; 2004.

2. Education ACfCM. Accreditation Council for Continuing Medical Education. ACCME Annual Report Data 1998; 2000.

3. Education ACfCM. Accreditation Council for Continuing Medical Education. ACCME Annual Report Data 2006; 2006.

4. Solomon DJ, Ferenchick GS, Laird-Fick HS, *et al.* A randomized trial comparing digital and live lecture formats [ISRCTN40455708]. *BMC Med Educ* 2004; 4: 27.

5. Bello G, Pennisi MA, Maviglia R, *et al.* Online vs live methods for teaching difficult airway management to anesthesiology residents. *Intensive Care Med* 2005; 31(4): 547–552.

6. Lockyer J, Sargeant J, Curran V, *et al.* The transition from face-to-face to online CME facilitation. *Med Teach* 2006; 28(7): 625–630.

7. Curran V, Lockyer J, Sargeant J, *et al.* Evaluation of learning outcomes in Web-based continuing medical education. *Acad Med* 2006; 81(10 Suppl): S30–S34.

8. Fordis M, King JE, Ballantyne CM, *et al.* Comparison of the instructional efficacy of Internet-based CME with live interactive CME workshops: A randomized controlled trial. *JAMA* 2005; 294(9): 1043–1051.

9. Ioannidis JP. Contradicted and initially stronger effects in highly cited clinical research. *JAMA* 2005; 294(2): 218–228.

10. Wyer PC, Allen TY, Corrall CJ. How to find evidence when you need it. Part 4: Matching clinical questions to appropriate databases. *Ann Emerg Med* 2003; 42(1): 136–149.

11. Randomised trial of intravenous streptokinase, oral aspirin, both, or neither among 17, 187 cases of suspected acute myocardial infarction: ISIS-2. ISIS-2 (Second International Study of Infarct Survival) Collaborative Group. *Lancet* 1988; 2(8607): 349–360.

12. Baker DW, Parker RM, Williams MV, *et al.* Use and effectiveness of interpreters in an emergency department. *JAMA* 1996; 275(10): 783–788.

# CHAPTER 8

# Teaching the intangibles: professionalism and interpersonal skills/communication

*David K. Zich, James G. Adams*
*Northwestern University, Feinberg School of Medicine, Northwestern Memorial Hospital, Chicago, IL, USA*

## Communication and professionalism

### Professionalism and communication in emergency medicine

At its core, professionalism is the ability to suspend self-interest for the benefit of patients and family and also for the effective management of the entire emergency department [1]. Physicians learn to suppress reactive instincts and emotions that are part of natural human response, especially during stressful events. Inherent in professionalism is commitment to honesty, proper use of the physician's authority, and an acceptance of accountability [1, 2]. Professionalism is a dynamic concept, one that requires self-reflection, especially during the formative stages, but additionally throughout one's career. Though the governing bodies of emergency medicine all agree that communication and professionalism are keys to medical training and practice success, little is offered about how to best teach and evaluate these skills [3]. This chapter will attempt to offer practical advice to emergency medicine educators.

*Practical Teaching in Emergency Medicine*, 1st edition. Edited by R Rogers, A Mattu, M Winters & J Martinez. ©2009 Blackwell Publishing, ISBN: 9781405176224

## Recommendation 1: provide motivation for professional behavior and improved communication

To effectively teach professionalism and communication skills, it is imperative to first outline the benefits for students.

1 Effective communication and professional behavior will enhance interaction, promote an accurate history and physical examination, minimize conflicts, and avoid distractions and misunderstandings. Effective skills will be beneficial every day of one's career.

2 No other medical concept will have as profound of an effect on the work environment, with the potential to enhance effectiveness, efficiency, coordination and teamwork. Conversely, ignoring these concepts can have extreme negative consequences on the above.

3 Proficiency in communication can serve as a powerful tool to
   a foster greater cooperation among consultants
   b improve the efficiency of the medical team [4]
   c increase the amount of information gathered from patient encounters
   d improve patients' understanding of their visit
   e increase patient compliance with the treatment plan
   f increase patient satisfaction with the physician
   g decrease lawsuits [5–8].

These skills will be essential for an effective and enjoyable career [9]. Being appreciated by patients and staff, feeling respected, and feeling rewarded by medical practice requires effective human interactions, marked by professionalism and communication skill.

## Recommendation 2: promote openness to continual growth

Once there is willingness to ensure professionalism and communication, self-reflection is required. Most doctors believe that they act professionally and communicate sufficiently well. Few are motivated to improve themselves. Barriers to enhancing professional behavior and effective interpersonal communication reside in deeply held attitudes, outlooks, personality traits, and developed habits. Personality traits are developed before medical school and residency but are also influenced during training. A great gift that academic faculty can provide is the encouragement to be open to continual development of communication and professional skills. Modeling such openness is ideal. The truly great physicians are on a lifelong quest for personal and professional growth.

## Recommendation 3: set expectations and establish standards surrounding the mission of emergency medicine

The trainee must understand that the specialty of emergency medicine is about caring for anyone at any time with varied conditions under variable circumstance. Patients come from the pinnacle of society and, more commonly, from the fringes. Acceptance of the mission to care optimally for all is essential. During the shift, negative judgment must be avoided. Development of the mindset of "unconditional positive regard" is helpful. It is not expected that the EP will accept all patient actions and behaviors, but the patient must always be considered worthy and must be viewed compassionately. The positive regard is contingent on nothing but humanity. Even as patients are counseled about harmful behaviors, if boundaries have to be set during ED care, or even when physical restraint is required, the actions should never be instituted as a punitive measure. All actions are in the interest of safety and sound care. The profession of emergency medicine is tasked to provide technically excellent care to all, under varied circumstance, with compassion. The trainee must embrace this mission in order for notions of professionalism to be understandable.

## Recommendation 4: observe, listen, evaluate and offer feedback

With standards and expectations set, teaching professionalism and communication can occur. During "apprenticeship" work in the ED, when learning is observational and participatory, role models are the dominant influence. When the role model offers insight and feedback, the trainee can improve. Experience alone, in the absence of feedback, can lead to overconfidence and perpetuate incorrect actions. Expertise is developed when effective feedback is provided. Teachers must be willing and able to model excellent behavior, observe behaviors of the trainees, and provide feedback.

In the real world, student learners will be exposed to both positive and negative role models [2]. In fact, 98% of medical students in six medical schools report witnessing unprofessional behavior by their faculty teachers [10]. Negative role models can be educational as well, provided the behaviors are recognized and discussed. Because of the frequency of observed negative behaviors, it is suggested that a discussion forum be provided for in-depth exploration of witnessed behaviors. The students can benefit from the wisdom of the teacher who facilitates this discussion. The department potentially benefits from the feedback provided by the students.

Deliberate positive discussions are also needed for the learner to reach a high level of performance. Given the extreme demands placed on emergency physicians during a typical clinical shift, it should not be assumed that student learners are noticing the positive keys to communication and professionalism [11]. If possible, emergency physicians should be aware that explicitly discussing challenging events and interactions can greatly aid those in training [2]. Having shifts where educators are present strictly to tend to the needs of the students, without patient-care duties, might help in deciphering positive and negative role model actions, and can also serve to evaluate student progress as well [12]. Other innovative methods of teaching include standardized patient encounters, high-fidelity simulations, and panel discussions, in addition to traditional didactic lectures [9, 13]. In reality, a combination of many of these modalities is required to teach the complexities of professionalism and communication most effectively.

Formal evaluation of communication skill is beneficial to ensure that observation and feedback occurs. Directly observed patient encounters are important to ensure that students are able to communicate effectively and compassionately. However, the best source of feedback can come from the patients themselves. A very carefully designed and validated tool for patient assessment of physician communication is provided to aid in physician development (see Table 8.1) [14].

## Recommendation 5: explicitly outline key components of a patient encounter, including the initial introduction, patient-centered interview, and concluding the visit

A common mnemonic for key components of a patient encounter is the SEGUE Framework checklist [5]. This stands for *S*et the stage, *E*licit information, *G*ive information, *U*nderstand the patient perspective, and *E*nd the interview. The mnemonic provides basic concepts.

**Table 8.1** Communication assessment tool survey used by patients to provide feedback to their physicians.

Communication with patients is a very important part of quality medical care. We would like to know how you feel about the way your doctor communicated with you. Your answers are completely confidential, so please be as open and honest as you can. Thank you very much.

| 1 | 2 | 3 | 4 | 5 |
|---|---|---|---|---|
| poor | fair | good | very good | excellent |

**Please use this scale to rate the way the doctor communicated with you. Circle your answer for each item below.**

| The doctor | poor | | | | excellent |
|---|---|---|---|---|---|
| 1. Greeted me in a way that made me feel comfortable | 1 | 2 | 3 | 4 | 5 |
| 2. Treated me with respectv | 1 | 2 | 3 | 4 | 5 |
| 3. Showed interest in my ideas about my health | 1 | 2 | 3 | 4 | 5 |
| 4. Understood my main health concerns | 1 | 2 | 3 | 4 | 5 |
| 5. Paid attention to me (looked at me, listened carefully) | 1 | 2 | 3 | 4 | 5 |
| 6. Let me talk without interruptions | 1 | 2 | 3 | 4 | 5 |
| 7. Gave me as much information as I wanted | 1 | 2 | 3 | 4 | 5 |
| 8. Talked in terms I could understand | 1 | 2 | 3 | 4 | 5 |
| 9. Checked to be sure I understood everything | 1 | 2 | 3 | 4 | 5 |
| 10. Encouraged me to ask questions | 1 | 2 | 3 | 4 | 5 |
| 11. Involved me in decisions as much as I wanted | 1 | 2 | 3 | 4 | 5 |
| 12. Discussed next steps, including any follow-up plans | 1 | 2 | 3 | 4 | 5 |
| 13. Showed care and concern | 1 | 2 | 3 | 4 | 5 |
| 14. Spent the right amount of time with me | 1 | 2 | 3 | 4 | 5 |

| The doctor's staff | poor | | | | excellent |
|---|---|---|---|---|---|
| 15. Spent the right amount of time with me | 1 | 2 | 3 | 4 | 5 |

The teacher can elaborate and share personal best practices for ensuring a successful encounter. Elaboration and reordering of steps are encouraged to improve upon this base.

For example, unlike the SEGUE checklist that suggests gaining an understanding of the patient perspective after all medical data is gathered, it is imperative that the physician attempt to gain this understanding before entering the room for the first time. This may be gleaned from the chief complaint and history provided by the triage process. The first few sentences spoken to a patient can determine the entire success or failure of the interaction. By attempting to gain the patient's perspective prior to the first meeting, physicians have the opportunity to create trust and favor while avoiding awkward miscues from an inappropriate affect upon entering the room. Successfully anticipating the emotions of patients and families is much more powerful than an initial generic approach. Naturally, that understanding will then refine and grow as the encounter progresses.

## The initial encounter, including introductions and physical contact

Powerful impressions are made during the first moments of the encounter with the patient. The patient makes an instinctive determination about whether the physician is trustworthy based on verbal and nonverbal cues. A key to success in establishing rapport with patients is to ensure an appropriate introduction. An offer to shake hands with everyone in the room should usually take place as part of the initial encounter. The patient should almost always be the first contact, even if incapacitated, to make clear that he or she is the primary focus of the physician. At some point during the interview a hand on the shoulder, the arm, or a pat on the lower leg can be comforting to many patients and further convey compassion and empathy from the physician. Though some people will mandate less intrusion of their personal space, appropriate, brief physical contact can create a tremendous humanistic connection between patient and provider. Mastering the initial encounter is a key task for the learner. This requires confidence and exposure to a variety of experiences with veteran physicians who facilitate the process through explicit instruction and role modeling.

## The "patient-centered interview"

Once introductions are established, information must be gathered. Creating an atmosphere that enables the patient to freely relate to the physician is critical. Even subtle differences in affect and attitude of the physician can have significant effect on how forthcoming patients are with their complaints. The following points will maximize the interaction and encourage the most information from patients [15].

1 Maintain proper, respectful eye contact with patients and family.
2 When appropriate, offer initial statements that show you understand their medical challenges.
3 Demonstrate kindness and concern. A warm smile or empathic facial gestures in response to information reinforces the patient's perception of the physician's interest. Verbal expression that you intend to provide thorough, expert care is appropriate, even when warm feelings of concern are absent.
4 Ask open-ended questions such as general queries that begin with "how" and "why." Questions encouraging yes or no answers or short replies limit the opportunity to gather important historical information.
5 Add facilitative rather than interruptive comments. Before interrupting or changing the topic, make sure that the patient's message is fully understood, since patients may have difficulty articulating the information or concerns.
6 Give patients the illusion that you have hours to spend with them while limiting the encounter to minutes. This takes skill and experience, but can be accomplished by
  a sitting during the interview rather than standing
  b using brief, tasteful interjections of humor when appropriate to the situation
  c tolerating short intervals of silence
  d accepting moments of non-medical conversation, demonstrating genuine interest in them as a person
  e listening deeply, to understand how the patient is coping
  f offering expressions of caring
  g providing appropriate reassurance.

Not only does the "patient-centered interview" tend to be more greatly appreciated by the patient, but also allows for a broader approach to differential diagnosis, protecting against prematurely focusing on an erroneous conclusion [3]. Included in this approach should be an inquiry as to what the patient is most concerned about. Too often patients will go through an entire encounter to discharge without specifically vocalizing their concern, such as whether they may have cancer, a sexually transmitted disease, or other issue. If not addressed, they may continue to believe their symptoms still represent a particular illness, and the main goal of seeking evaluation was not met.

## Closing the initial interview

After the initial interview is complete, there are important issues to cover with the patient: (1) a discussion of possible diagnoses; (2) an explanation of the tests necessary to narrow the focus; (3) how long, approximately, the patient can expect to be in the ED; and (4) any treatment necessary in the interim. It is imperative that this discussion be carried out in layperson terms. It is acceptable and even encouraged to use medical terminology, provided an explanation follows in simplified language.

## Concluding the visit

Once all the data has been gathered, concluding the visit involves four main steps:

1 Explaining test results.

This requires great skill in translating medical data to layperson terminology. Essential to any discussion should be the degree to which a test is abnormal as well as the limitation of the test. For instance, an "abnormal ECG" may mean non-specific findings that are unchanged from their previous ECG, to ST elevations of an acute MI. Placing the ECG findings into context for the patient, including what needs to be immediately addressed, addressed sometime in the future, or requires no further action, is important. In addition, informing the patient of the test's limitations, such as the fact that significant heart disease may still exist despite minimal changes on an ECG, is critical.

2 Providing a diagnosis when possible or exclusion of pathology when appropriate.

Many of the diagnoses given to patients are of little consequence to their lives and may not require much effort from the physician's standpoint. Conversely, delivering catastrophic results to patients or families such as newly diagnosed cancer or the death of a loved one obviously takes great care and skill. In-depth discussion of effectively delivering life-altering information is beyond the scope of this chapter. However, simply recognizing the impact a diagnosis may have on a patient is a key initial step. Each encounter requires the provider to adapt the approach to the individual circumstance. A miscarriage may be a relatively minor occurrence to a young patient with an undesired pregnancy, or could be devastating to a childless couple who have been trying to conceive for years. The diagnosis of a sexually transmitted disease may not only be a lifelong affliction, but could also result in the end of a marriage if it reveals infidelity. No matter how many times the physician has seen an illness, it is imperative to remember that this may be the first time the patient has been told of it, and what has become blasé for the provider may be life altering for the patient. Though all diagnoses should be delivered with compassion and empathy, the amount of time spent with the patient will need to be adapted based on the patient's circumstances and response. Correctly, anticipating and adjusting the delivery of information based on the patient's perspective is imperative when communicating results.

In addition, given the limited resources and time of an emergency physician, exclusion of serious pathology is often all that can be accomplished. Patients may leave the department disappointed that a firm diagnosis has not been established. Setting expectations in the initial interview may help to mitigate against this at the end of the encounter, but frank discussion about the role of the emergency department in medical evaluation is sometimes necessary. When appropriate, plans for continued evaluation should be made.

**3** Relaying the plan for treatment, future testing, and further evaluation.

Whether or not the diagnosis is certain, laying out a concrete plan for a patient is essential. An effective plan not only takes into account medical necessity, but also special physical and emotional needs of the patient. It should encompass alleviation of symptoms, appropriate follow-up, and reasons to seek emergency care again. Communicating this in layperson terms is essential, and ideally should be followed by a confirmation that patients have understood the directions. Written instructions should accompany the verbal explanation when summarizing the key points.

As an adjunct to all but the most simple of plans, an explanation as to why the chosen approach is in the best interest of the patient should be given. Most physicians assume that any instruction they give to patients will be interpreted as in their best interest, and explicitly detailing the benefits is a waste of time. However, often the final plan is different from a preconceived idea the patient may have had prior to seeking treatment. Typical situations involve patients who believe they are in need of an antibiotic, a radiologic test, or even admission to the hospital when the medical indication does not exist. When they do not get what they believe is necessary, patients may assume the care provider is incompetent, has a personal dislike towards them, or may even have secondary gain from denying them. Careful, compassionate explanations as to the benefits of the chosen plan as well as the hazards of the alternatives will help to allay these misconceptions. For instance, patients should not only be told the clinical reasoning behind why an antibiotic is not indicated, but the hazards of side effects and allergic reactions that make it against their best interest to get the prescription. Radiological tests that are not indicated should be described in relation to the radiation dosages to which patients are exposed, and the remote but real association with future malignancy. In addition, for those desiring unnecessary admission to the hospital, a discussion of the interrupted sleep patterns, often less than desirable food, and exposure to in-hospital pathogens should be presented as reasons why the benefits do not outweigh the risks of admission in this case. In other words, every plan should be framed as the optimal choice in a set of options that provides the maximum benefit with the minimum risk to the patient.

**4** Explaining uncertainty that may remain.

Discussing diagnostic uncertainty with patients can be as important as explaining a diagnosis itself. A job of the caregiver is often educating patients on the inexact nature of medical science. Certainly, some diagnoses are unequivocal such as a displaced long-bone fracture. However many others have a particular degree of uncertainty. In these cases it is imperative to relay to the patient the ambiguity of the results, as well as the next steps to ensure optimal care and further clarification. Great skill is required to help the patient to differentiate between a rational, scientific approach to an uncertain diagnosis from mere guessing. The key is to convey limitations inherent in any test results without implying limitations in the provider's ability. The axiom "cautiousness in diagnosis, confidence in plan" should be kept in mind when talking with patients and family.

5 Eliciting questions.

Finally, patients should be given ample opportunity to ask questions. Crucial to the success of this step is appearing unhurried and open to inquiry. At this point, patients are often exhausted, overwhelmed, and continue to be intimidated by their care providers. Leaving with unanswered questions decreases patient compliance and therefore leads to worse outcomes. Anything that can be done to promote questions is encouraged. Such steps include staying seated when eliciting questions, directing the inquiry to family as well, and repeating a call for questions after each one is answered.

## Recommendation 6: recognize the importance of communicating well with nurses

Time spent in communication with nursing is usually second only to communication with patients and family. The student must be taught that effective two-way dialogue is essential for the most efficient and safe patient care [4]. Motivation arises not only from the critical role nursing plays in the delivery of medical services, but also from the fact that they typically spend a much greater amount of time with the patient than does the physician. As a result, they may provide details of a patient's history that were not given to the physician or relay important background information that aids greatly in relating to patients or family before entering the room. Nurses act as a final safeguard for physician orders and can aid in detecting inappropriate doses of medications or allergies that may have been overlooked. Nurses are also in a prime position to detect subtle changes in patient status and alert physicians to intervene before problems become too critical.

Points to emphasize to students and young physicians are these: Treating nurses with respect and understanding can increase nursing performance and make the physician's job easier. If physicians discourage nursing input, they will not get it, thereby limiting a valuable resource that can increase their liability in the end. Nurses do not have the same level of training and experience as physicians and should not be expected to provide the same comprehensive levels of data or insight, but this should not lessen the value of what is relayed. In short, collegial, professional relations with nursing will encourage their input, thereby helping physicians work more efficiently, protect them from liability, and improve their overall quality of care.

## Recommendation 7: frame the approach to communicating clearly, respectfully, and confidently with consultants

Communicating with consultants provides unique challenges as well. Teaching successful navigation through a typical encounter requires the student to understand the underlying situational dynamics. Though this is considered a peer-to-peer interaction, essentially emergency physicians have the upper hand, as they are the ones delegating work or responsibility to their consultants. Though consultants usually are aware that they are on-call, consults from the emergency department are unplanned events that always interrupt another activity whether this is sleep, a social event, or a professional obligation. Emergency physicians who understand the frame of reference of their consultants will be much more successful enlisting their expertise.

There are several critical issues to the interaction to be taught to the student:

1 Often by simply acknowledging the disruption to their day, consultants become more receptive as colleagues.
2 Emergency physicians can further engage consultants by appealing to their sense of pride and duty. Expressing that their expertise is required to help and care for a patient and giving a brief explanation as to the limits reached in the care thus far can add to the motivation.
3 While providing an understanding and appreciation of the consultants' abilities, emergency physicians must maintain their status as the care provider in charge. To maintain respect from the consultant's position, emergency physicians must be well prepared with a clear understanding of the clinical scenario as well as any data that supports a call for a specialist.

**4** Care should be taken to avoid the misconception that one physician is being called upon to help another physician. Rather the conversation should always be framed as two physicians that are joining efforts to help the patient.

**5** Thank the consultant for their time and expertise.

## Recommendation 8: be the role model of professionalism in words and deeds

For the patient, every person is important. The student, trainee, attending physician, nurses, technicians, and others influence their anxiety and confidence with the care. Healthcare is mysterious and frightening to the patient and family. The off-handed jokes that are overheard, a too-casual style of dress, a disinterested and dismissive manner can, alone or in combination, impair trust. It is easy to forget how sound travels in a busy emergency department, and a single derogatory comment overheard by the patient outside of their room can undo all of the good rapport that the provider has built up with that patient. While individual care giver's personal styles, manners and preferences may be respected, there are limits. As a rule, if the manners, dress and behaviors do not enhance the trust of the patient, they are probably not acceptable.

## Recommendation 9: discuss the importance of acknowledging the good work of others

Those who work in the emergency department labor under challenging conditions and work hard, with great skill, to meet patient's needs. The stresses are palpable; the difficulties are at the forefront of our attention. It is typical to take for granted the excellent behaviors that are present. Observing and mentioning the good behaviors will positively reinforce them. Students should be encouraged to regularly observe and verbally recognize good behavior of fellow physicians, nurses, and support staff members. If every attending physician made this effort, the mood, morale, and ultimately the productivity of the department would elevate.

## Remediation of students having difficulty with professionalism and communication

Just as the subject of professionalism and communication is extremely complex so are the various ways that a student can fail to progress in proficiency with these important skills. The approach to remediation depends largely on the reason behind the failure to progress. There are three main groups of people who have difficulty learning the subject:

1 The willing student who has difficulty comprehending or grasping the concepts
2 The willing student who is emulating the wrong role models
3 The unwilling student who, for whatever reasons, rejects the concepts

Remediation of the first group may benefit most from supervised simulated patient encounters. Watching how the student responds to various scenarios, followed by a brief discussion of how an experienced emergency physician would respond, will help the learner begin to develop an approach to a variety of situations.

The second group of students may best be served by direct observation by a dedicated educator during a given period in the ED, free from clinical duties. Active discussion about positive and negative role models can help to guide the student in the right direction.

The third group often represents the most challenging students to remediate. However, showing the students the consequences of poor communication and lack of professionalism often serves as the best motivator for change. This can best be accomplished by time with the quality assurance branch of the department, addressing patient complaints and negative patient outcomes. Accumulating a case file of legal settlements against ED physicians nationwide can serve as excellent studies in the subject. The student should be expected to identify communication strategies with the patients, families, ancillary staff, and outside physicians that could mitigate against adverse situations. In addition, it is imperative to point out how professionalism, or lack thereof, can help or exacerbate the situation.

Finally, perhaps no other area of medical competency is as sensitive an indicator for the existence of troubling personal issues. For those students demonstrating severe deficiencies in professionalism and communication, educators must be vigilant for signs of depression, substance abuse, and other strains of student life. Often, rapid and aggressive intervention might be necessary to correct deficiencies of these core competencies when problems stem from underlying psychiatric disorders or addiction.

## Conclusion

The environment in which emergency physicians must function is full of challenges and potential barriers to effective patient care.

A comprehensive understanding of communication skills and professionalism is critical to a successful and rewarding career. Teachers must first create the motivation to learn, and then provide a global approach to conveying these complex concepts. If successful, this knowledge will lead to respect and admiration by patients and peers alike, enriching interactions on professional and personal levels throughout life.

### Summary points

1. Provide motivation for professional behavior and improved communication.
2. Promote openness to continual growth.
3. Set expectations and establish standards surrounding the mission of emergency medicine.
4. Observe, listen, evaluate, and offer feedback.
5. Explicitly outline key components of a patient encounter, including the initial introduction, patient-centered interview, and concluding the visit.
6. Recognize the importance of communicating well with nurses.
7. Frame the approach to communicating clearly, respectfully, and confidently with consultants.
8. Be the role model of professionalism in words and deeds.
9. Discuss the importance of acknowledging the good work of others.

### Helpful tips

1. A learner should always be observed directly in patient encounters at least once a shift.
2. A learner should always observe the teaching physician during a patient encounter at least once a shift.
3. Be aware of teaching moments during interactions with nurses, ancillary staff, and consultants.
4. Be aware of negative role models and how they are affecting the learner.
5. If the teaching physician encounters a particularly difficult patient or situation, understand these are the most valuable teaching opportunities to talk through during or soon after the encounter.

# References

1. Finkel MA, Adams JG. Professionalism in emergency medicine. *Emerg Med Clin North Am* 1999; 17(2): 443–450.
2. Kenny NP, Mann, KV, MacLeod H. Role modeling in physicians' professional formation: reconsidering an essential but untapped educational strategy. *Acad Med* 2003; 78(12): 1203–1210.
3. Rhodes VR, Vieth R, He T, *et al*. Resuscitating the physician–patient relationship: emergency department communication in an academic medical center. *Ann Emerg Med* 2004; 44: 262–267.
4. Spencer R, Coiera E, Logan P. Variation in communication loads on clinical staff in the Emergency Department. *Ann Emerg med* 2004; 44(3): 268–273.
5. Hobgood CD, Riviello, RJ, Jouriles N, Hamilton G. Assessment of communication and interpersonal skills competencies. *Acad Emerg Med* 2002; 9: 1257–1269.
6. Oh J, Segal R, Boal J, Jotkowitz A. Retention and use of patient-centered interviewing skills after intensive training. *Acad Med* 2001; 76: 647–650.
7. Smith RC, Lyles JS, Mettler JA, *et al*. A strategy for improving patient satisfaction by the intensive training of residents in psychosocial medicine: a controlled, randomized study. *Acad Med* 1995; 70: 729–732.
8. Laidlaw TS, Kaufman DM, Macleod H, Sargeant J, Langille DB. Patients' satisfaction with their family physicians' communication skills: a Nova Scotia survey. *Acad Med* 2001; 76(10, Oct RIME suppl): S77–S79.
9. Totten VY, Ethics and teaching the art of emergency medicine. *Emerg Med Clin North Am* 1999; 17(2): 429–441.
10. Green M, Zick A, Makoul G. (2007) Professionalism assessment tools based on patient, nurse, and physician perspectives. Powerpoint presentation, publication pending, Feinberg School of Medicine, Northwestern University, Chicago, IL.
11. Gisondi MA, Smith-Coggins R, Harter PM, *et al*. Assessment of resident professionalism using high-fidelity simulation of ethical dilemmas. *Acad Emerg Med* 2004; 11(9): 931–937.
12. Reisdorff EJ, Hughes MJ, Castaneda C, *et al*. Developing a valid evaluation for interpersonal and communication skills. *Acad Emerg Med* 2006; 13(10): 1056–1061.
13. Cydulka RK, Emerman CL, Jouriles NJ. Evaluation of resident performance and intensive bedside teaching during direct observation. *Acad Emerg Med* 1996; 3: 345–351.
14. Makoul G, Krupat E, Chang CH, *et al*. Measuring patient views of physician communication skills: developing and testing of the Communication Assessment Tool, *Patient Educ Couns* 2007, doi:10.1016/j.pec.2007.05.005
15. O'Mara K, Communication and conflict resolution in emergency medicine. *Emerg Med Clin North Am* 1999; 17(2): 451–459.

## SECTION 3
# Teaching Specific Groups

# CHAPTER 9
# Teaching medical students

*David E. Manthey*
*Wake Forest University School of Medicine, Medical Center Boulevard, Winston-Salem, NC, USA*

## Why teach medical students?

It is July 1st in the emergency department (ED) and we are all wondering about the start of the new physicians-in-training because we have no idea of their knowledge base or their abilities. They do not seem to understand what to do outside of their own specialty. Do not blame them: ask yourself why you did not do a better job of teaching them as students.

All physicians-in-training were once medical students. Students make their decision upon which specialty to enter based on their interactions with faculty, what they observe while on rotation, and their perception of that specialty. We can affect all three of these facets and attract the best students to our own specialty by setting a professional and competent clinical example that they would want to emulate. We can also teach the student what our specialty does in the total realm of care for the patient. In the same light, all the physicians that enter specialties other than our own also come from medical students. Therefore, we have a tremendous opportunity to impart the abilities and limitations of our specialty to students entering other specialties so that they can better understand how our two specialties can work together for the benefit of the patient.

The medical student's opinion about yourself and how you handle patients will help with your rapport with them when they become physicians. If treated with respect, given responsibility and taught while on service, their opinion of our specialty may just be more

*Practical Teaching in Emergency Medicine*, 1st edition. Edited by R Rogers, A Mattu, M Winters & J Martinez. ©2009 Blackwell Publishing, ISBN: 9781405176224

favorable down the line. One of the most compelling reasons to teach medical students may be that you or your family will one day need the services of one of these medical students turned specialists – should not you help them with both the desire and the ability to be the best doctor they can be?

From the ED standpoint, this is a clear opportunity to explain to them that no matter what specialty they enter, they will deal with an emergency physician for one of their patients, friends, or family members. Therefore, they need to know how we work and what we do. Patients are seen based on their acuity. All patients who present to the ED will be seen, no matter the hour, insurance status, or degree of illness, but some might have to wait. This also means that we have a limited time to spend with each patient. We are sometimes forced to make decisions about care without the luxury of knowing all the history or all of the test results. It is also important that they know that their patient will be well cared for when sent to the ED.

## What is so unique about emergency medicine (EM)?

As most students do their rotations in EM during their fourth year, I will point out the uniqueness of the rotation based on this perspective. These students have completed their core inpatient rotations where most patients already have a diagnosis and treatment plan established. Because of this, many students are not familiar with the approach to a patient with an undifferentiated complaint or how to develop a list of differential diagnoses.

On the wards, students are expected to gather an all-encompassing history and perform a detailed physical examination and then describe the treatment of all of the identified problems. In the ED, students are expected to evaluate an undifferentiated patient and perform a focused complaint oriented history and physical examination to identify a case specific differential diagnosis and case management plan. All of this occurs within perhaps 15 minutes. We expect them to independently present an evaluation and treatment plan, often with minimal time to consult a textbook or obtain direction from a physician-in-training.

On the wards, most patients have already been stabilized and if not, the students are never really independently in charge of the patient's care. But in the ED, we often allow students to provide supervised care to potentially sick patients, not just from the standpoint of the vital signs, but in terms of time sensitive items such as myocardial infarctions and strokes.

On other services, the student can expect to see types of patient or complaints specific to that service. For example, on an orthopedics rotation, the student will see fractures and musculoskeletal injuries and while on cardiology, they will see diseases isolated to the heart. They can concentrate on a relatively smaller realm of information (from the medical student's point of view) than in the ED. In the ED, the student may see a patient with chest pain, then a patient with a fracture, then a two-day old with fever all in one day. We ask the student to synthesize all the information they have gained in the core clerkships and apply it to each patient encounter.

We ask students to perform procedures that they had little exposure during their entire third year. In fact, we seek them out and then send them in with little preparation. We assume that they know how to do the procedures; how else would they have made it to the fourth year? We assume that the student must have learned suturing on Surgery and Obstetrics rotations, but in reality, they were given the educational opportunity to learn.

## What are the problems unique to EM?

On the wards for four, six, or eight weeks, the student often works with the same physicians. They get to learn all of the quirks of their supervisors and nuances of what to say or do on rounds to stay out of trouble. In the ED, they have limited continuity with a single attending and each attending has different expectations of both the student and the care of a specific disease.

Upon arriving to the EM rotation, many students have a preconceived notion of what EM can offer them. We can use this opportunity to give them a better understanding of our specialty and what we have to offer patients. The student will see a wide variety of patients in the ED. This aspect of not knowing what you might see next may be part of the thrill of being an EM physician, but it can be unnerving to many students.

EM rotations are often a mandatory fourth year rotation so many students are not in the department by choice. Some of them will take this time to improve their knowledge base, see things they will never get a chance to see again based on their specialty choice, or learn how to take care of medical and surgical emergencies. Others will bide their time by hiding until the rotation is over. Taking the time to know the student's specialty choice and helping them see patients and diseases that they will one day care for may develop a rapport with the student.

## Qualities of an effective teacher

As this topic is covered in many other sections of this book, I will offer only a few relevant pearls. Students respond better if you treat them with respect. Acknowledge their presence. Know their name and what specialty they have chosen. Engage them in conversation about something other than the patient.

Maintain a professional behavior. Derogatory language about a patient, nurse, or other service is inappropriate and will diminish the student's regard for you and your specialty. Disrespectful treatment of staff or patients will do the same. One of the hurdles of EM is overcoming the often incorrect perceptions that other services have of us. Treating other services with disrespect in front of students or other staff damages our credibility and makes overcoming this hurdle even more daunting.

Show clinical competence in your field. Remember that many students have already been taught a certain approach to a disease and when we alter that approach, confusion as to who to believe may arise. Take the time to show the student the literature that supports your practice, explain why you differed from what they have been taught or what the consultant expected, and acknowledge that there is often more than one way to treat a disease.

Teach with enthusiasm because it is infectious. Anger, cynicism, rudeness, and disrespectful behavior breed the same in your student and that disrespectful behavior might be directed at you one day. Your teaching ability has a positive and significant effect on the student's learning [1].

## Teaching philosophy

A good teacher should remember several things about the adult learner. Developing an intrinsic motivation in the student is much better than imposing an extrinsic motivation. Motivating the student by showing that an improved knowledge base makes you quicker (because you do not have to look it up), allows you to ask the right questions (because you know what points are important in the history), and maintains the respect of the patient (because you did not have to go ask) is a much longer lasting motivation than telling them it will be on the test.

Aim for a higher level of cognition than just the accumulation of facts. Knowing to use beta-blockers as first line therapy for aortic dissection is not as important as knowing to decrease the shearing force and not just the blood pressure. That is why nitroprusside is not used first or alone.

Information should be filtered into a structured format for use in future clinical scenarios; this can be done by teaching a general rule [2]. The statement that young adults with back pain do not usually need radiographs is true. The statement that red flags for needing further radiographic evaluation include cancer, fever, trauma, previous surgery, neurological deficits, intravenous drug abuse, etc. allows the student to apply that knowledge to a wider range of patients.

Determine the student's level of ability and knowledge base before you start to teach. Each student has a different level of knowledge and experience. Ask probing questions to see where their knowledge base ends so that you know where to start teaching. Otherwise you may deliver a great talk on kidney stones to someone who just finished urology. It is still a great presentation but it is not needed or appreciated by the student. Knowing their abilities allows you to give the student a little more (or less) independence in their clinical decision-making. Finding gaps in their knowledge base also allows you to identify areas for self-directed learning, such as having them look up Well's criteria in the diagnosis of pulmonary embolism.

## Educational objectives and curriculum

Any clerkship should structure the educational experience around a set curriculum based on obtainable and defined learning objectives [3]. The clerkship should provide both a learning environment to increase the student's knowledge as well as provide an opportunity to gain clinical experience and skills. An Educator's Guide and Curriculum Guide are both available to the reader [4, 5].

Feedback is crucial to effective teaching and is reviewed in greater detail in another chapter of this text. If you do not provide feedback, you are in essence reinforcing the student's current behavior. Specifically identify areas of strengths that you want the student to continue and areas of weaknesses that they can work on. This is easiest to do when you allow them to develop a presentation, differential diagnoses, and evaluation plan instead of doing it for them. They quickly learn that if they stall for a mere few seconds, most faculties will step in and tell them what to do.

Promote reflection in the student by encouraging them to self evaluate. Students are often harder on themselves than you will ever be. If they identify a problem that you agree with, their self-awareness followed by your acknowledgement and plan for correction will lead to a stronger desire for change and monitoring of the behavior [6]. If it is a knowledge deficit that is identified, the student will have the desire to fill the void and not just answer the question.

## Clinical teaching

When applied to teaching medical students, structure for the administrative aspects of a rotation will allow the student to adapt quickly to the new environment with less anxiety and stress. This allows them to learn more and ask more clinically oriented questions. Guide the student in their selection of patients to help them to stay within the limits of their ability. Allow them sufficient, not excessive, time to complete a directed history and physical examination. Allow them time to review the records and develop their presentation. When the clinical situation does not afford the student this time, explain to them that you are going to guide the case quickly due to the status of the department or the patient.

Understand that the presentation of the case is the prime focus of the student–faculty interaction. This is the student's time to shine and their level of anticipation/anxiety will match that. As presentations in the ED are more concise and directed, inform the student of what you expect from them during the presentation. The best solution would be if every faculty could agree on a single format and this format be given to the student at orientation to the rotation. When the student presents the case to you, allow them to finish without interruption.

If you have no expectations of the student, they will meet them easily and often do no more. Therefore, expect the student to develop a list of differential diagnoses. This list should include the more common diseases as well as those diseases that cannot be missed without a significant morbidity or chance of mortality to the patient. Expect them to use the history and physical to remove, retain, or order various diagnoses on the differential. Ask them to defend this final list, as it will allow you insight into their thought process as well as identify their level of knowledge on the subject. This allows you to know what to teach and what to encourage them to read.

Expect them to generate an evaluation plan for the patient which includes why they are recommending a specific test (lab, radiograph, and physical exam) and what they will do with the results. Stepping over them and telling them what to order may allow you to move the patient along faster but it does not allow you to assess their knowledge base or correct any misconceptions such as ruling out infection because of a normal white blood cell count.

Debrief a student at the end of a clinical interaction so that you can address the student's performance and agree upon the student's knowledge level, clinical competence, and interpretation of the history, physical, and clinical data [7]. Further feedback will follow after more clinical encounters, but directed discussion at the end of a single encounter allows for reinforcement of clinical findings, rules, and thought processes. The clinical experience allows the student a framework upon which further reading/learning can be built. The student will more quickly remember information that is associated with a clinical scenario than one that is based solely on unattached reading.

Be prepared to teach when the moment arises. Teaching in the clinical arena is a fluid process. Remain committed to teaching, even if it is only in 30 second blocks of time at the end of a case. Take advantage of "teachable moments" and specifically inform learners that you are teaching them something. Faculty, who have only one standard way of teaching, will limit the opportunities to teach. Instead, learn various different ways to teach at the bedside (discussed in Chapter 4) including the microskills model, the one-minute observation, learner-centered precepting, and modeling problem solving [8]. Having a variety of teaching skills and the desire to teach allows the faculty the ability to identify many more teaching opportunities and the ability to adapt the teaching to the clinical environment at that time. Some days allow for longer and more in-depth discussions. Some busy shifts and more difficult patients lend themselves to modeling the thought process and patient interaction skills. Remember that you do not have to teach after each patient encounter or during each student interaction as your time, ability and mood may not allow for it. As well, the student's level of knowledge and ability may not require additional teaching, just feedback on a job well done.

## Techniques to prevent the student from being overwhelmed or overwhelming you

Orientation is important to the student's ability to adapt to the new environment and lays the ground work for the limitations on what they will be allowed to do. Setting a limit of carrying no more than three active patients at any one time takes the undue pressure of too many patients off of the timid student and stops the eager student from picking up every patient in the department.

Structure their learning experience so that they know how to attend to the administrative details of the department, such as how to document charts, how to use various computers and programs, and how to order labs and radiographs. Describe the ED approach to them so that they realize why we ask them "Sick or Not Sick?" and why they should request our help immediately for the sick patient. Explain the need for resuscitation before the evaluation is completed. The ability to make decisions with limited information is the cornerstone of a good EM physician, but well beyond the ability or experience of an average medical student. Again, guide the student in their selection of patients to help them stay within the limits of their ability and your desired level of input.

Reassure students that they will not be alone in the care of the patient. Inform the overly confident student that you will be providing close oversight and that all management decisions should be cleared with you before implementation. Provide the timid student the safety net that if they let something fall between the cracks, you will be there to catch it. Remind them that their priority is learning. This may be by reading on a topic or by seeing an interesting finding on another patient.

By introducing the student to the interesting patients and findings (ECG, radiograph, and physical exam) in the ED, you allow the student to view a wide variety of disease without specific patient care responsibilities. You get a breather, and they gain knowledge. It also increases the chance that they will see patients with the less common disorders or presentations.

## Summary points

1. Expect students to develop a differential and treatment plan. Assess their level of knowledge to know where to start your teaching.
2. Do not tell students the diagnosis or what to order unless you explain your thought process out loud so they can see the steps you took to get there.
3. Teach general rules that can be used in future clinical scenarios.
4. Do not think you have to teach on every patient. Each day is different depending on you, the student, and the clinical scenario.
5. Promote learner autonomy by letting students perform self-evaluation. Points they identify will be more vigorously corrected than ones you identify.
6. Teach students pearls that are clinically relevant instead of those that are germane only to trivia buffs and written tests.

# References

1. Stern DT, Willians BC, Gill A, *et al*. Is there a relationship between attending physicians' and residents' teaching skills and students' examination scores? *Acad Med* 2000; 75: 1144–11
2. McGee SR, Irby DM. Teaching in the outpatient clinic: practical tips. *J Gen Intern Med* 1997; 12(2): S34–S40.
3. Ende J, Pozen JT, Levinsky NG. Enhancing learning during a clinical clerkship: the value of a structured curriculum. *J Gen Internal Med* 1986; 1: 232–237.
4. Coates WC. An educator's guide to teaching emergency medicine to medical students. *J Acad EM* 2004; 11(3): 300–306.
5. Manthey DE, Coates WC, Ander DS, *et al*. Report of the Task Force on National Fourth Year Medical Student Emergency Medicine Curriculum Guide. *Ann Emerg Med* 2006 March; 47(3): e1–e7. Epub 2006 February 1.
6. Branch WT, Paranjape A. Feedback and reflection: teaching methods for clinical settings. *Acad Med* 2002; 77: 1185–1188.
7. Kelly AM. Getting more out of the clinical experience in the emergency department. *Emer Med* 2002; 14: 127–130.
8. Alguire PC, DeWitt DE, Pinsky LE, Ferenchick, GS. Case based learning. In: *Teaching in Your Office: A Guide to Instructing Medical Students and Residents*. Philadelphia: American College of Physicians–American Society of Internal Medicine. ISBN 1-930513-07-0, 2001: 43–65.

# CHAPTER 10

# Teaching trainees from other services in the emergency department

*Michelle Lin*
University of California San Francisco, San Francisco General Hospital,
Emergency Services, San Francisco, CA, USA

## Introduction

Academic emergency departments (ED) are staffed by Emergency Medicine (EM) trainees and by trainees from various other departments. Many Residency Review Committees (RRC) in the United States under the Accreditation Council for Graduate Medical Education (ACGME) require that their trainees have clinical exposure to EM during their postgraduate training years. The ED provides unique clinical experiences and learning opportunities, relevant to various postgraduate training programs. Programs with such a mandate include internal medicine, pediatrics, and anesthesia. Additional programs within other fields also electively schedule an EM rotation for their trainees for the unique educational experiences [1].

Off-service trainees typically spend only 2–12 weeks each in the ED during their entire training period. It is during this brief time that they immerse themselves in learning, understanding, and practicing the principles of EM and acute care medicine. These principles include immediate assessment, intervention and stabilization, treatment, and diagnostic planning. These are pivotal skills, which will be immediately applicable in managing their specialty patients with acute medical complaints. Furthermore, non-EM trainees within the United States oftentimes serve as field physicians for

*Practical Teaching in Emergency Medicine*, 1st edition. Edited by R Rogers, A Mattu, M Winters & J Martinez. ©2009 Blackwell Publishing, ISBN: 9781405176224

international expeditions, missions, and medical facilities. It is thus crucial for EM educators to appropriately teach these practitioners of EM in both the domestic and the global arena of health care.

## Advantages to having non-EM trainees

Just as off-service trainees benefit from an EM rotation, the ED benefits from the presence of off-service trainees. First, regardless of whether the ED has an EM training program or not, academia-affiliated EDs are typically busy and are in need of extra health care providers. This is especially true on EM trainee conference days, when all EM trainees are excused from weekly clinical duties to attend didactic sessions. Under the supervision of board-certified emergency physicians, off-service trainees function almost as EM trainees. In a study comparing ED quality indicators on conference days versus nonconference days, there was no difference in the numbers of diagnostic tests, consultations, unscheduled return visits, or patient satisfaction. Off-service trainees, however, had longer decision-to-admit time (333 minutes versus 313 minutes for EM trainees) and length of stay for admissions (490 versus 445 minutes for EM trainees) [2]. Furthermore, having off-service trainees to help with staffing may allow for shorter trainee shifts, such as 8- or 10-hour shifts. This may reduce trainee fatigue and improve overall group morale.

The ED also benefits from the presence of off-service trainees through team-building. Although the concept of team-building is less tangible than staffing numbers and shift hours, building a sense of camaraderie and spirit of collaboration between the EM trainees/attendings and the off-service trainees often have positive, long-lasting effects when the EM trainees/attendings need to consult from or admit patients to various services. The off-service trainees are no longer receiving calls from impersonal voices on the telephone but rather from colleagues, who they know, have worked with, and trust.

## Models for teaching off-service residents

The wide spectrum of ED patients naturally provides a wealth of learning opportunities for trainees. On a day-to-day basis, there is an unpredictability of patient presentations, which translates into trainees receiving variable experiences during their EM rotation. It is impossible to guarantee that each trainee will encounter a checklist of chief complaints and perform a set list of basic procedures. In an ideal EM rotation with unlimited time and resources, off-service trainees would be provided supplemental learning opportunities, to help ensure a more uniform educational experience for each trainee.

Currently, EM rotations employ various didactic approaches. On one extreme, some rotations provide no didactic teaching at all for off-service trainees. On the other extreme, EM rotations provide off-service trainees with a separate lecture curriculum, designed specifically for them and to which they are relieved from clinical duties during those dates. Unfortunately, no single educational model is applicable to all EDs. In general, successfully educating the off-service trainee requires a combination of bedside teaching along with either informal or formal didactic lectures. Each of these methods has advantages and disadvantages.

## Bedside teaching

Bedside teaching is the primary modality employed in the ED to teach trainees while on-shift. With growing emphasis on competency-based outcomes for learning, bedside teaching provides the greatest opportunity to directly assess and improve learner competency. Other major advantages of this educational model include the fact that teaching is tailored to each trainee's expertise and knowledge level. Furthermore, teaching is directly relevant to active patient care issues. The learners can then receive immediate feedback providing them with insight into their strengths and deficiencies.

There are challenges to implementing an off-service curriculum based solely on bedside teaching. The primary challenge is that using only a bedside teaching model leads to a nonuniform educational experience. Teaching becomes based on the daily spectrum of patients. Furthermore, off-service trainees often only rotate in the ED for 2–12 weeks during their entire residency training. Thus, they may experience an extremely variable clinical experience and quality of education in the ED. Furthermore, their EM rotation experience is influenced by the ED type (community, academic, county, and/or trauma center), patient demographics, and census volume.

An additional challenge of using bedside teaching is having attending physicians, who are untrained in performing effective bedside teaching. Bedside education is a less structured, less tangible, and less predicable teaching method than, for instance, giving a PowerPoint lecture. Another growing challenge is the increased clinical demands on attending physicians from ED overcrowding and thus less time for direct learner observation and supervision. Chisholm *et al.* found that during a resident's ED shift, only 3.6% of it involved an EM attending directly observing him or her conducting direct patient care [3]. Without adequate time available for attendings to observe the trainee, instituting a culture of bedside teaching and feedback is extremely difficult.

## Informal didactics during a shift

In EM rotations at some institutions, off-service trainees are excused from clinical duties for 15–60 minutes daily to attend a structured educational session. These sessions can be case-based discussions, chart reviews, skills workshops, or informal mini-lectures. This concept is modeled after teaching sessions in other departments, such as "morning report" or "noon conference."

There are three major advantages to this informal didactic teaching approach. First, these sessions provide daily protected times, dedicated to teaching those who are on-shift. Second, these sessions help to ensure a more consistent and a broad foundation of learning regarding common ED presentations, treatment plans, and management dilemmas. Finally, providing a basic foundation of knowledge to the off-service trainees allows for more advanced teacher–learner discussions. Less time is spent on learning the fundamental facts with more time spent on sophisticated discussions.

The disadvantages to this teaching approach as the sole educational model for off-service trainees include the attending physicians not being able to directly assess each trainee's examination skills, interpersonal and communication skills, and real-time decision-making abilities. Furthermore, it is difficult for the attending physician to tailor teaching to each trainee's knowledge level, since the discussion group has learners at different stages of training.

Two major obstacles toward instituting informal didactic sessions revolve around patient care staffing issues and attending availability. First, overwhelming patient care responsibilities and insufficient resources may preclude trainees from being released from the clinical area, even for a brief period of time. Second, the attending physician on-shift may not have time to conduct informal didactics because of patient care responsibilities. Similarly attending physicians, who are not on-shift, may be too busy with other academic responsibilities. The faculty, as a whole, would have to determine if their time is worth investing in these daily educational sessions, since faculty resources and time are often limited.

## Formal didactics

Lecture-based curricula typically exist in most academic EDs. Because most EM rotations do not have the resources to run a curriculum dedicated purely for off-service trainees, some EM rotations release their off-service trainees from clinical duties to participate in one of the existing curricula. One advantage to this educational approach is that the off-service trainees are extra learners within an already existing lecture series. No additional teaching resources are needed. The didactic sessions can provide at least a more broad foundation of knowledge for off-service trainees. Formal teaching sessions may minimize the frequency and the total time spent by attending physicians repeatedly teaching fundamental concepts on an individual level.

Several disadvantages exist with using formal didactic sessions as the sole form of off-service trainee education. The main disadvantage is that the lecture material in the EM residency and the medical student lecture series may be too EM-focused. An additional challenge lies in releasing the off-service trainees to attend didactic sessions. Because EM residents are required to attend the weekly conferences, the ED becomes only staffed by EM attendings, mid-level providers (if available), and off-service trainees on those dates. Many EDs cannot function without the off-service trainees helping to offset the deficit in health care providers on those lecture days. Often it is easier to release off-service trainees to the medical student lecture series, which may be more appropriate in some cases. For instance, a pediatric intern may have the same knowledge level as a senior medical student regarding non-pediatric related topics, such as vascular ultrasonography.

Another challenge to implementing formal didactic educational opportunities for the off-service trainees includes the competing obligations such as their longitudinal clinics and their own department conferences. Furthermore because the EM rotation is shift-work-based and has circadian dysrhythmias, oftentimes lectures may be coincidentally held on days when the off-service trainee has either a day off or has just completed an overnight shift. In these instances, they may not be as inclined to attend formal didactic lectures, making it difficult to ensure them a consistent didactic educational experience.

## Practical tips to improve models of teaching

There is no single, best-answer solution to teaching off-service trainees in the ED. Each institution will have to balance the available resources in the ED, faculty time and availability, and needs of the off-service trainees.

### Practical tips: being a more effective bedside educator

With a growing emphasis on outcomes-based assessment and competency in medical education, bedside observation, teaching, and feedback will likely play an increasingly greater role in the ED. For off-service trainees, there are two unique considerations that should be taken into account. First, off-service trainees have a variable knowledge base within different aspects of EM. These trainees may be more junior or senior in training. Their medical specialty may have minimal or significant overlap with EM. For instance, a transitional intern entering a dermatology residency may not have as strong an EM knowledge as a categorical third-year resident in internal medicine, who is about to enter a cardiology fellowship. Bedside education should be tailored to each learner. The second consideration is that off-service trainees only rotate through the ED for 2–12 weeks during their entire medical training period. During this time, their educational goals focus on acquiring knowledge and skills that are not taught in any other rotation. Box 10.1 provides

---

**Box 10.1** Examples of educational objectives and goals for off-service trainees

1. Learn how to the work-up an undifferentiated patient.
2. Learn how to manage common orthopedic injuries and complaints.
3. Learn how to lead a resuscitation and implement Advanced Cardiac Life Support algorithms.
4. Learn how to approach airway management.
5. Recognize common and uncommon presentations of medical and traumatic emergencies.
6. Understand classic toxicologic syndromes and emergencies.
7. Obtain proficiency in performing procedures, such as phlebotomy, peripheral and central venous line placement, wound closure, and splinting.

a list of typical educational objectives and goals that off-service departments often wish their trainees to achieve during their EM rotation.

Understanding these unique challenges for off-service trainees can help bedside educators become more effective. In two surveys, which asked accomplished EM educators and ED learners what qualities best characterize a skilled bedside educator, many common themes were found. Table 10.1 lists the combined findings from these two studies with specific suggested strategies for teaching off-service trainees [4, 5]. These bedside education principles should not consume the attending physicians' time in the ED, but rather help them focus and maximize quality time toward imparting concise, high-yield teaching points. If practiced on a daily basis, the culture of bedside education becomes more routine, streamlined, and second nature.

**Table 10.1** Practical strategies to help EM faculty improve bedside education in the ED, specifically for off-service trainees [4, 5].

| Strategy to improve bedside education | Specific strategies for off-service residents |
| --- | --- |
| 1 Agree on expectations for the ED shift | Spend 1–2 minutes at the beginning of the shift to ask trainee about their background training level and learning goals for that shift and the rotation overall. |
| 2 Demonstrate a good teacher attitude | Be approachable and maintain a mutual level of respect. |
| 3 Actively seek opportunities to teach | For interesting cases, share teaching points with the entire ED team so that other trainees can learn from the cases. For any shift, come prepared with a list of 10–12 high-yield talking points that are relevant for off-service trainees (e.g. missed foreign bodies in wounds, aggressive fluid resuscitation in septic patients, addressing the most emergent causes of chest pain before assuming the patient has esophageal reflux). |
| 4 Tailor teaching to learner and situation | Use teachable moments well, teach concise points relevant to the trainee's educational goals, respect time constraints, and/or ask how the trainee would have managed a similar case in clinic. |

*Continued*

| Strategy to improve bedside education | Specific strategies for off-service residents |
| --- | --- |
| 5 Optimize faculty–learner interaction | Tailor supervision based on the trainee's skill level, encourage active learning, and solicit the trainee's thoughts on patient care plans rather than dictating the plan from the start. |
| 6 Provide real-time feedback | Immediately after completion of a task or before the ED shift ends, spend 1–2 minutes to provide positive comments and constructive formative assessments of the trainee's medical knowledge, oral presentation, decision-making capabilities, and/or procedural competencies. |
| 7 Use additional learning resources | Strategies include teaching residents high-yield online resources, procedural technique using models, radiology interpretation skills using databanks of images, and specific topics by assigning a publication article to read. |
| 8. Be a role model and demonstrate useful ED skills | Professional modeling occurs every day with trainees learning by direct observation of attendings interacting with patients and staff, multitasking in a busy clinical setting, and dealing with stress. |
| 9 Improve the learning environment | Find a more isolated area in the ED to give feedback comments, especially if they are constructive, and make teaching points. |
| 10 Learn formal teaching techniques from faculty development programs on bedside teaching and providing feedback | Faculty development programs, workshops, and textbooks exist to help attendings learn more formally about bedside teaching and feedback techniques. |

Bedside teaching can only succeed, however, if there is an infrastructure in place. With less time for ED attending physicians to observe residents and conduct bedside teaching and feedback, some institutions have recently implemented a novel innovation of a "teaching attending" on-shift, whose sole responsibility is to observe, teach, and provide formative feedback to learners in the ED. This allows the clinical ED attending on-shift to focus almost entirely on patient care and patient flow issues, because a large portion of the bedside educational responsibilities has been transferred to the teaching attending [6].

## Practical tips: enhancing the didactics component

There should ideally be a didactic educational component to supplement bedside education for off-service trainees. It serves to build a more consistent educational experience for all the rotating off-service trainees from month to month. Didactics, however, does not necessarily mean a formal lecture series. Although EM conferences and medical student series are viable educational options for off-service trainees, short, daily (or even weekly) teaching sessions in the ED also can serve as informal didactic experiences. These sessions can occur, for instance, immediately following morning sign-out rounds, when the ED is traditionally less busy, or during the mid-day when there are more learners in the ED. These sessions can be taught by either the attending physician on-shift, the "teaching attending" on-shift, or an attending assigned to teach the session. Teaching topics could be cycled every 1–3 months and would highlight high-yield EM topics, keeping in mind the common learning objectives for off-service trainees (Box 10.1).

Didactics can also be moved completely outside of the ED. Attending physicians can teach common EM topics at large-group educational sessions held by other departments. For instance, one can teach suturing and wound care at a few large-group workshops at the beginning of the training year to minimize the number of individual suturing workshops needed in the ED. Similarly, resuscitation techniques and common ED pitfalls can be taught to more senior trainees in a single setting before they rotate in the ED.

Alternatively, in addition to moving education away from the ED, education can move away from live interactions. Teaching can be done at the learner's own pace and time using the Internet. With web-based technologies becoming more advanced and playing an increasingly important role in medical education, didactics may be provided in the form of online educational modules and online discussion forums. Online educational modules would ideally be interactive, use multimedia, and enlist an EM faculty member, whom trainees could contact if they had questions. These modules, for example, could include teaching videos on basic procedures or an approach to undifferentiated patients categorized by chief complaint. Online discussion forums may also be employed but require a significant faculty facilitation presence to ensure content accuracy, reinforce teaching points, and encourage active discussions. Without active facilitation, the discussions may lose momentum, and residents may quickly lose interest in this learning modality. When done correctly, however, online discussion forums can be a significant teaching tool for all trainees in the ED. This form of asynchronous learning allows all trainees, regardless if they are on-shift or off-shift, to post comments, answer questions, and address discussion points.

## Conclusion

Off-service trainees play a crucial role in the ED, both as providers and as learners. EM rotations provide various educational experiences for the trainees, ranging from none to a heavy didactic and bedside teaching component. Teaching is dependent on the available resources in the ED, faculty time, and trainee needs. Typically successful programs include a combination of bedside education, informal didactics while on-shift, and formal didactic sessions. Although educating off-service trainees is often seen as lower educational priority in the department after EM trainees and medical students (who may potentially be future EM trainees), these trainees should not be relegated to pure "work-horses" of the EM rotation. Many of the bedside teaching and feedback skills for EM trainees and medical students are easily applicable for off-service trainees. Efforts to optimize teaching in the ED at the bedside, at the whiteboard, in a conference room, or on the Internet will benefit all learners in the ED. It is important not to forget that off-service trainees belong in this pool of learners.

---

### Summary points

Off-service trainees in the ED are often a peripheral educational focus, because they are not pursuing a career in EM. Because patients within their specialty, however, often present with acute problems during their outpatient visits or inpatient stays, it is crucial that these trainees also learn and understand the basic EM approach to assessment, intervention and stabilization, treatment, and diagnostic strategies for these patients. This learning should occur within the ED at least in the form of skilled bedside education and scheduled on-shift didactic activities, such as daily morning teaching rounds. If greater resources and technological capabilities are available, more structured off-site didactics and asynchronous online discussions, respectively, should be incorporated into the training curriculum.

## Pitfalls

**1** Off-service trainees should not be treated as mere workers within the ED. They deserve an EM education, similar to EM trainees and medical students.

**2** Do not assume that learning expectations from the non-EM trainee are the same as the EM trainee or medical student. Ask the non-EM trainee what he/she would like to learn at the beginning of the shift, and seek out relevant learning opportunities from the trainee's own or other trainees' patient cases.

**3** Bedside teaching should not be burdensome for the educator or the non-EM trainee. Do not overwhelm the learner with endless teaching points related to a patient's care. Effective bedside teaching can take as little as one minute, by tailoring teaching to the learner's knowledge base, giving comments in real time, and creating a respectful, nonthreatening learning environment.

**4** Do not schedule on-shift, teaching rounds on an elective basis or nonperiodic cycle. Set routine times for teaching rounds and strictly adhere to them. This will require buy-in and consensus amongst the ED educator group to ensure sustainability and successful implementation of these rounds.

## References

1. Accreditation Council for Graduate Medical Education. [Internet]. Chicago, IL; c2000–2007. Available from: http://www.acgme.org/. Accessed September 30, 2007.
2. French D, Zwemer FL Jr., Schneider S. The effects of the absence of emergency medicine residents in an academic emergency department. *Acad Emerg Med* 2002; 9(11):1205–1210.
3. Chisholm CD, Whenmouth LF, Daly EA, Cordell WH, Giles BK, Brizendine EJ. An evaluation of emergency medicine resident interaction time with faculty in different teaching venues. *Acad Emerg Med* 2004; 11(2): 149–155.
4. Bandiera G, Lee S, Tiberius R. Creating effective learning in today's emergency departments: how accomplished teachers get it done. *Ann Emerg Med* 2005; 45(3): 253–261.
5. Thurgur L, Bandiera G, Lee S, Tiberius R. What do emergency medicine learners want from their teachers? A multicenter focus group analysis. *Acad Emerg Med* 2005; 12(9): 856–861.
6. Shayne P, Heilpern K, Ander D, Palmer-Smith V. Protected clinical teaching time and a bedside clinical evaluation instrument in an emergency medicine training program. *Acad Emerg Med* 2002; 9(11): 1342–1349.

## CHAPTER 11

# The education of resident physicians in emergency medicine: A United States perspective

*Stuart P. Swadron, William K. Mallon*
Los Angeles County/USC Medical Center, Keck School of Medicine of the University of Southern California, Los Angeles, CA, USA

## Teaching resident physicians

The relationship between emergency medicine (EM) faculty and their residents is unlike the one that exists with medical students or residents from other primary specialties. This closer, long-term relationship becomes the cornerstone of the residents' clinical practice skills and patterns. When EM faculty members are working together with residents within their program, they are not contributing to or augmenting the training of future physicians, they are providing its foundation.

The learning that takes place in an EM training program is bidirectional. Residents and their faculty become very familiar with one another during the course of a three- or four- year program and have the opportunity to gain an in-depth knowledge of each others strengths as learners and teachers, respectively. This also allows for a much more complex learning process that builds upon shared experience.

## EM residency infrastructure and support

### The residency office: a hub of activity and a myriad of relationships

The residency office interacts with multiple individuals and agencies within a complex environment (Figure 11.1). Some of these parties

*Practical Teaching in Emergency Medicine*, 1st edition. Edited by R Rogers, A Mattu, M Winters & J Martinez. ©2009 Blackwell Publishing, ISBN: 9781405176224

function as academic or administrative overseers (e.g. Dean's Office, Chair, Graduate Medical Education Office), whereas others can be viewed as constituencies (e.g. the residents and the faculty). Because the residency office is accountable to so many parties whose objectives are often divergent, a program director must possess very strong interpersonal skills. He/she must be perceived as conciliatory and reasonable (someone that people would naturally go to for guidance during a conflict) to gain credibility and currency within the institution. It is necessary to be both a leader, and, at times, a follower, as part of a larger Graduate Medical Education (GME) community. The respect and support of those who provide oversight to the residency office is a critical prerequisite for the success of a residency training program. Without it, it is impossible for the residency office to advocate for those things necessary to advance the program.

The residency office must also be resourced properly to achieve its goals. The workload of the residency has periods of greater intensity throughout the year (e.g. interview and recruitment season, the orientation of new residents), and periodically throughout the accreditation cycle (e.g. internal reviews, Residency Review Committee – Emergency Medicine (RRC–EM) site visits). There must be enough flexibility within the department to devote extra resources during these times. Lack of administrative support for the residency office faculty is a common concern among program

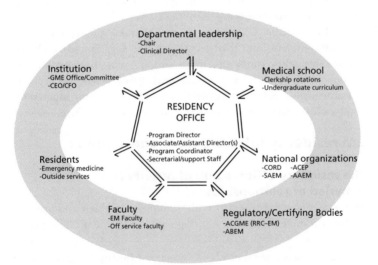

**Figure 11.1** The myriad relationships of the residency office.

directors, and along with a resultant lack of academic productivity, has been cited as a negative influence on program director longevity. In a recent survey of program directors in EM, inadequate protected time for scholarly activity, a lack of a career/family balance, and insufficient time overall to do the job required were the most commonly cited problems in their position [1] (Table 11.1).

## Continuity of leadership

Because the average program director's tenure is relatively short (median of five years [1]), many residents will experience a change in leadership during their training. It is thus very important that some continuity be maintained, usually through the succession of another faculty member already involved in the residency office. In the most recent national survey, it was found that 92% of program directors have an assistant or an associate program director and that most new directors have previously served in this capacity prior to their appointment. Whereas some have actively sought the role, many have felt obligated to assume it after a resignation of the previous director. In fact, 24% reported that they had accepted the position because no other suitable candidate was available.

**Table 11.1** Most common concerns cited by program directors in emergency medicine.

| Problem | Likert score Average* | Standard deviation |
| --- | --- | --- |
| Lack of adequate time to do the job required | 3.46 | 1.23 |
| Career needs interfere with family needs | 3.39 | 1.22 |
| Lack of adequate faculty help with residency matters | 3.09 | 1.17 |
| Budget concerns for support of residency activities | 3.25 | 1.29 |
| Inadequate release time for scholarly activity | 3.28 | 1.30 |

* Scale of 1 to 5. All other potential problems scored less than 3.
Beeson *et al.* Characteristics of emergency medicine program directors. *Acad Emerg Med* 2006; 13(2): 166–172. With permission from Wiley-Blackwell.

The complexity of the residency office and the multiple relationships that it must foster both locally and externally make it essential that the program director and the assistant director be thoroughly familiar with the residents, key people within the institution, and the program's accreditation status. To that end, an apprenticeship model is appropriate, with the aim of always having faculty within the program (and preferably with the residency office) who intend to assume the program director position.

## Scheduling and its effect on learning

Scheduling of both residents and faculty has a potential to make a tremendous impact on education. Although the Accreditation Council for Graduate Medical Education (ACGME) duty hour regulations have done much to eliminate the exhausted resident from patient care areas, less has been done to delineate and encourage scheduling strategies that can positively affect teaching and learning.

Fundamentally, teaching requires energy from both the learner and the teacher. Conflicting with this is the obvious reality of 24 hour/7-day care – and in EM, both residents and faculty must provide service throughout the night. Multiple authors have looked at circadian rhythm disruption in the workplace and have suggested techniques to minimize "night shift" effects, but few residencies have integrated these concepts into their schedule. Core sleep preservation (a fixed sleeping period) and forward phase shifting (e.g. a day shift/evening shift/night shift sequence) both serve to decrease circadian rhythm disruption and improve energy levels for teaching and learning [2, 3].

Shift durations for both faculty and residents generally range between 8 and 12 hours (the maximum allowed by the RRC–EM). Whereas residents may prefer 12-hour shifts to maximize their days away from the hospital, it is likely that a shorter shift duration is more optimal for learning. In our program, faculty shifts are generally shorter than resident shifts, and they are staggered. We try to schedule the residency office faculty on a swing shift that overlaps evenly with two separate resident shifts. This provides an excellent opportunity to maximize the frequency of their exposure to all of the residents (Figure 11.2).

## Dedicated teaching shifts

When it is actually quantified, the time that residents interact with their faculty during clinical shifts is very limited. At one large urban

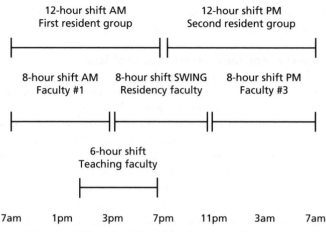

**Figure 11.2** A model for scheduling of faculty and residents.

program, mean total interaction time was 20% of the shift duration, with only 3.6% spent with the faculty member directly observing the resident in action [4]. To address this reality, some programs have introduced dedicated teaching shifts (teach-only faculty shifts), to assist the faculty member designated as the attending staff on duty. When these shifts are assigned to faculty members with demonstrated ability and experience as EM teachers, the learning environment is immediately enhanced [5]. The attending staff on duty is now freer to attend to patient safety and flow issues, whereas the "teaching attending" can maximize opportunities for learning. A teaching attending can also provide more thorough supervision of individual patient encounters and procedures. And lastly, they can provide better detailed real-time evaluation and feedback – facilitating future learning while completing the required documentation of these activities to fulfill RRC–EM requirements.

Although not all programs have the luxury of additional faculty hours to provide teaching shifts, even a limited number of four to six hour shifts at strategic times (e.g. peak volume hours), can go a long way toward improving the teaching milieu in a program. Excellent performance on resident feedback surveys can be used as a criterion to select faculty members for such shifts, providing an incentive for excellence in bedside teaching. One important caveat for programs employing this model is to ensure that a clear delineation exists between the two attending staff physicians in terms of responsibility for clinical decisions – typically the teaching attending does not assume clinical responsibility except for procedures being supervised, and the attending staff on duty must still review and approve of the management of all of the patients in their assigned clinical area.

## Residency program culture and conflicts

The overall morale and culture of a residency program is critical because it affects the learning of every resident in the program. Although different programs have their own style with respect to protocol and hierarchy, one hallmark of a successful program is a healthy degree of resident leadership and involvement. Residents invest a tremendous amount of themselves into their housestaff years, and many are motivated to help set the course for their own training. There should be opportunities through the department's GME Committee or other institutional committees and work-groups to get involved. For many, this will serve as an opportunity to explore a career in academic medicine or future leadership roles within the community.

There are many benefits of involving residents in the administration and planning of the training program. In addition to the critical need for the resident perspective on issues related to their own training, the sense of ownership created makes for more satisfied and committed learners, less distracted by the common nuisances and irritants of residency training. It should also be borne in mind that despite the successful introduction of duty hour limits, residency training is still demanding – physically, academically, and emotionally. Being attentive to what residents tell us and being mindful of their wellness is a responsibility that is shared by the entire faculty.

A key conflict exists between service and education during residency training. Although these two components of postgraduate training are not necessarily mutually exclusive, ultimately, residency programs are regulated by the ACGME, which considers residents to be learners first. Over time, residency training has transformed from being largely akin to an apprenticeship to a more formal, structured educational program. Nonetheless, residents understand that there is a service component to their training, and they are no less motivated than the faculty to ensure the efficient operation of the department. Imbalances in the service/education ratio may be more apparent in some areas of the emergency department (ED) than in others and during off-service rotations. The best way to deal with this reality is to have a policy of openness and transparency with regard to the clinical needs of the department, and to provide a mechanism for feedback and improvement so that educational objectives are met.

Another eternal conflict exists between resident autonomy and patient safety. Although faculty members appreciate the need for residents to have sufficient autonomy to develop clinically, they often worry that too much autonomy will come at the expense of patient safety. Although these two ideals will always exist in some sort of dynamic equilibrium, they are not necessarily incompatible. A common complaint heard from residents about faculty members is that they can be inflexible about patient management. Faculty members should consider making changes to a resident's management plan only if it is dangerous, allowing residents to practice in a safe, but not completely controlled, supervisory environment.

Assurance of sufficient resident autonomy extends far beyond their relationship with individual faculty members. It is the responsibility of residency office to provide an environment where residents are supervised, and also make autonomous clinical decisions and perform their own procedures, especially during critical resuscitations. If the department of EM lacks sufficient influence at the institutional level, especially in a training institution with large training programs in surgery, anesthesiology and critical care, it may be very difficult to create the environment necessary for this autonomy to exist. Nevertheless, ensuring patient care access and decision-making responsibility is absolutely critical for the success of the program.

## The core competencies

The six core competencies were mandated to be integrated into U.S. residency training programs in 2001 as the first phase of the ACGME Outcome Project [6]. Although the eventual objective of the project is to improve the quality of GME through the measurement of educational outcomes, the initial phase has served mostly to provide a common nomenclature for the process of evaluation. In fact, most of the instructional tools and the assessment techniques that were subsequently described to address the six competencies were in use prior to the Outcome Project. The six core competencies, as well as the tools used to teach them and assess them, are outlined in Table 11.2.

For most EM faculty not directly involved in residency administration, three of the six competencies, patient care, medical knowledge, and interpersonal skills and communication, are self-explanatory. The remaining three, professionalism, practice-based learning and improvement, and system-based practice, are not as obvious, and all have been defined specifically in relation to EM.

## Systems-based practice

System-based practice has a very central meaning in EM. To be considered proficient in system-based practice, a resident must "demonstrate an awareness of and responsiveness to the larger context and system of health care and the ability to effectively call on system resources to provide care that is of optimal value"

**Table 11.2** The ACGME core competencies.

| Competency | Teaching | Assessment |
|---|---|---|
| Patient care | Lectures, particularly those that are case based | In-service exams |
| | Internet or CD learning | CORD exams |
| | High-fidelity simulation | Med-challenger-based quizzes |
| | Procedure labs | SDOT |
| | Critically appraised topics | Simulation |
| | | Home-based exams |
| | | End-of-rotation evaluations |
| | | OSCE or standardized patients |
| Medical knowledge | Lectures (traditional or case based) | In-service exams |
| | Small-group instruction | CORD online Question Bank |
| | Morning report case conference | Homegrown examinations |
| | CD or online instruction | • Ultrasound interpretation |
| | Journal club | • ECG interpretation |
| | Assigned readings | • Core-content area |
| | Models and simulators | Mock oral assessments |
| | | Direct observation |
| | | Standardized direct observation |
| | | Models and simulators |
| | | Portfolios |

*Continued*

| Competency | Teaching | Assessment |
|---|---|---|
| Communication and interpersonal skills | Resident portfolio<br>Resident retreats<br>Lectures on skills<br>Evaluation as teaching tool<br>Faculty model behavior<br>Simulated cases | Direct observations<br>360-degree evaluations<br>Global assessment<br>Curtain evaluations<br>Consensus evaluation |
| Professionalism | Didactic curriculum | Written examinations of knowledge, principles, and policies |
| | Case-based discussion | Computer-based or oral exams with embedded ethical issues |
| | Clinical ED experiences encompassing patient management, with application of ethical principles to clinical situations | OSCEs with standardized patients |
| | Visually based teaching tools (CD-ROMs, videotapes, Internet-based teaching educational programs) | Modified essay questions |
| | Colloquial settings and retreats | Direct observation and SDOT |
| | | 360-degree evaluation |
| | | ACGME toolbox: self-administered rating forms and psychometric instruments |
| System-based practice | Administrative rotation | Bedside evaluations |
| | Out-of-hospital care (EMS) rotations | SDOT |
| | Departmental and hospital committees | Resident portfolios |
| | Patient follow-up | 360-degree evaluations (nursing, peer, ancillary staff) |

*Continued*

| Competency | Teaching | Assessment |
|---|---|---|
| | Case write-ups | Standardized oral exams with issues involving consultants, interpreters, resources |
| Practice-based learning | Evidence-based medicine reviews of clinical questions | Direct feedback on the conclusions drawn by the resident in a journal-club conference |
| | Journal clubs | Feedback from the CAT conference |
| | Critically appraised topics | Critical assessment of the resident's periodic portfolio summaries |
| | Attending CQI meetings | Critical assessment of the resident's M&M conference summaries |
| | Self-assessment of portfolio | |
| | Resident-led M&M conferences | |
| | Mentoring by faculty | |

CD = compact disc; CORD = Council of Residency Directors; OSCE = objective structured clinical exams; ACGME = Accreditation Council for Graduate Medical Education; CAT = critically appraised topics; CQI = continuous quality improvement; M&M = morbidity and mortality; SDOT = standardized direct observation tool.

Stahmer *et al*. Integrating the core competencies: proceedings from the 2005 Academic Assembly consortium. *Acad Emerg Med* 2007; 14(1): 80–94. With permission from Wiley-Blackwell.

[7]. Whereas this competency may play a more secondary role to patient care in other specialties, in EM, expertise within various systems is easily as important as individual patient care. From the very beginning to the very end of each shift, the emergency physicians (EP) is operating within a set of complex, overlapping and interconnected systems: the prehospital system, trauma, cardiovascular, neurologic, and other specialized care systems, the institution's on-call specialty consultation, diversion, and surge capacity systems. Decisions made in the care of individual patients impact the care of all other patients in the department. Every decision to pursue a specific assessment or a treatment plan is done so within the context of prioritization and the differential application of a finite set of resources to all of the patients in the department. Moreover, safe and efficient disposition from the ED requires the highest level

of sophistication and understanding of the entire health care system beyond the ED – both its inpatient and outpatient components.

Although various tools have been proposed for the teaching and the evaluation of systems-based practice, none, in our view, is as important as real-time assessment and direct observation within the clinical area. This can be done by multiple evaluators: faculty, peers and colleagues, nursing and ancillary staff, as well as the residents themselves. Supervising faculty in our program are asked to assess EM residents during clinical shifts in real time with respect to their ability to efficiently multitask, delegate, supervise, and interface with the many individuals and systems that they encounter. They are also asked to comment on the cost-effectiveness of their utilization of departmental resources.

## Professionalism

Professionalism appears to overlap with interpersonal and communications skills, however, there are certain specific skills and behaviors critical to the practice EM that underscore proficiency in this competency. Some can be assessed in the clinical setting, when observing the handling of patient care transfers (sign out), negotiation of ethical dilemmas, and difficult patient encounters. Others can be evaluated outside of the clinical realm, such as compliance with medical record keeping and the multiple, recurrent administrative requirements of residency training. In our program, a component of the professionalism evaluation of is now completed by the residency coordinator, who assigns a score to each resident. This score is based on their responsiveness to administrative queries from the residency office, integrity in shift trading, fulfillment of teaching responsibilities, timeliness, and overall reliability. Although some of this assessment is necessarily subjective, much of it is easily quantifiable with clear and consistent record keeping.

## Practice-based learning and improvement

Practice-based learning and improvement is the critical review of one's own clinical work and the growth that occurs as a result of that review. Activities related to evidence-based medicine, such as literature searches and journal clubs, as well as peer-review activities, such as chart reviews and quality assurance audits, fall under this competency. Perhaps the most important process in practice-based learning for EP is patient follow-up. It is difficult to prevent recurrent mistakes and bad habits if one does not regularly follow-up with patients and their providers. The RRC–EM specifically requires a formal process documenting regular follow-up on a selection of patients seen in the ED. Although there are different ways of implementing this requirement, it is critical that follow-up occurs by some formal mechanism. Invariably, the information gleaned through following cases to their outcomes touches on other competencies, especially patient care, medical knowledge, and systems-based practice. We require a simple regular follow-up exercise on a selection of patients from different areas of the department (e.g. major trauma, fast track, etc.), both admitted and discharged home.

## Clinical teaching paradigms for EM faculty

### Effective teachers in a chaotic environment

Several Canadian authors have examined the unique learning environment of the ED and attempted to quantify the relative importance of specific faculty attributes and teaching strategies [8–11]. Several key themes consistently emerge in their interviews and surveys of EM residents and well-recognized EM teaching faculty. As a prerequisite to teach, teachers need not know everything, however, the residents must have confidence that they have a mastery of the core curriculum in EM. They must also bring a positive and an enthusiastic attitude to the clinical area. The most effective teachers spend more time listening and becoming familiar with the resident: their strengths and weaknesses, their educational needs, their knowledge base, and their specific understanding of each specific case. They are also able to work around the well-known challenges in EM teaching (department crowding, time, and patient flow demands) and even turn these challenges into opportunities. For example, when multiple patients present simultaneously, the faculty member might perform triage themselves, explaining their rationale as they go to the more junior members in the department. An effective teaching method is thus employed (teaching by example) that exploits a unique opportunity in the ED (a multi-casualty scenario), without compromising patient safety. Effective teachers seize on good cases and teaching situations when they occur to benefit all of the learners in the department, and lastly, they give feedback constructively and consistently.

### Matching approaches to patient flow and acuity

Although specific methods for bedside teaching are described in other sections of this book, little has been written on the actual mechanics or structure of resident teaching in the ED. Probably the most important variables that determine how teaching takes place are patient volume and acuity. Other factors, such as the number of trainees on-shift simultaneously and their postgraduate year level, are obviously important as well.

During very slow times in the department, when there are no patients waiting to be seen, it may actually be possible to gather the entire team to do bedside rounds. When the department is moderately busy, either a one-on-one patient rounding technique or a small group technique may be utilized, with the faculty member mindful of minimizing disruption to patient flow. Teaching can be synergistic with patient flow rather than antagonist. Practically speaking, this means that specific actions taken and questions addressed during faculty–resident interaction time are directly related to the patient care tasks that need to be completed, rather than a discussion tangential to the patients at hand. During such "work rounds," the faculty member can also help the resident by getting a task or two completed for them (e.g. checking lab values) to remove some of the time pressure that can impede learning during a busy shift.

One of the key rate-limiting steps in patient management that makes junior doctors slower is medical decision-making or "what to do next" in patient management. One technique that takes advantage of this fact is especially useful in a lower acuity area, where a lot of patients are being seen simultaneously and treatment plans need to be made quickly. Residents and other learners (medical students, mid-level providers) all pick up a chart and quickly assess their respective patients in a short time frame (e.g. 10 minutes). The team then makes a quick round of all of the patients together, and after a very brief presentation and formulation, the faculty and team helps the presenter to finalize their management plan. During these quick working rounds, all of the learners benefit from having to consider the management of each others' cases, as well the collective wisdom of the entire group, under the leadership of the faculty member. This process can be repeated several times during a shift, but there needs to be significant intervals between sessions to give residents time to complete tasks and operate efficiently without interruption.

The busier and more chaotic a department becomes, the more "teaching by example" becomes a modality of choice. Faculty can model their understanding of systems-based practice by skillful triage, marshaling of departmental and extra-departmental resources,

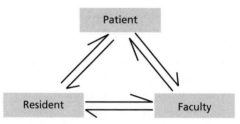

**Figure 11.3** The residency education triangle.

and timely decision-making. In reality, as senior residents approach the final interval of their training, they often serve in this role themselves – and in many programs a heavy emphasis is placed on their ability to do so.

## The residency teaching triangle: pursuing educational "Nirvana"

As Sir William Osler said over 100 years ago, "take [the student] from the lecture room, take him from the amphitheatre … put him in the outpatient department, put him on the wards … no teaching [should occur] without a patient for a text, and the best is that taught by the patient himself" [12]. "Educational nirvana" occurs when a resident with the appropriate foundation encounters a patient or a scenario that they have not encountered before, preferably requiring a treatment or a procedure that they have not yet performed, with an enthusiastic faculty member acting as a catalyst in the learning process (Figure 11.3). As a catalyst, the faculty member should allow the patient to do the teaching whenever possible, as Osler taught, but he/she can enhance the process by reinforcing the key features of the presentation and/or clinical decision-making that need to be recognized for future encounters.

As a resident proceeds through residency and gains more experience with different clinical presentations, occurrences of "educational nirvana" will occur less frequently. Nonetheless, there will still be important subtle presentations of common, life-threatening illnesses that will imprint upon their clinical expertise – every opportunity to emphasize these moments should be taken, as well. Because an important rate-limiting step in the resident clinical teaching triangle is the patient and their pathology, the ideal patient population for a training program is one that is varied and rich with pathology. No teaching tool or technique can substitute for this.

## Pattern recognition/visual diagnosis

In EM, pattern recognition and visual diagnostic skills are particularly important. Rapid determination of a treatment plan requires the rapid generation of a differential diagnosis – and in a large number of cases this is done by simple pattern recognition. Moreover, when an experienced clinician is able to recognize such patterns effortlessly, it can be quite frustrating for a resident who is unable to draw from a comparable database of experience. Commonly, junior residents will ask "how could I be expected to figure that out?" or "will I ever be able to pick things like that up?"

Whenever important patterns are recognized or good visual stimuli available, every opportunity should be taken to share them with other residents and students in the department at that time. By no means does this mean that the department must come to a standstill for a group lecture or a bedside session; the patient can simply be pointed out to the other residents, or a quick trip to the relevant bedside could occur at the beginning of their working rounds. It also may be possible to capture visual stimuli such as imaging studies, ECGs, photo and/or a video clips (with appropriate patient consent) for later use in a conventional conference setting. We make frequent use of digital video recording to capture critical findings, and to review procedural technique. Video recording has also been used to document entire resuscitations for later critical review, particularly in major trauma cases. Although this practice has been reported to be very helpful from a quality improvement and a practice-based learning perspective, it involves some medico-legal and ethical concerns that some feel preclude its routine use [13].

## Encouraging knowledge retention

Although advances in the field of educational theory do not generally make their debut in the realm of GME first, there are some ideas and techniques that have arisen from cognitive science that are relevant to bedside teachers in the ED.

Getting residents to integrate new information into their existing fund of knowledge can be a challenge. A common refrain among residents is "I've already forgotten that three times, I'll never remember it!" Information is often more easily assimilated when it is added to an existing foundation – something that junior residents, in particular, are just developing. When too much new information is presented at once, it is likely that little of the knowledge will be retained.

One mechanism for enhancing retention is to formally link new information gleaned at the bedside to existing knowledge.

Once the faculty member knows what the resident's existing base of knowledge is on a given subject, the new information can be attached to that existing knowledge. Simply by asking, "what do you know about this?" and then linking a new piece of knowledge to that existing data, the odds of retention increase.

Because memories appear to last much longer when they are reinforced in a timely manner after their initial creation, residents should be strongly encouraged to bring at least one new idea or question from each shift home with them for supplemental reading. This will ensure a more lasting impact and a mental bridge to the clinical experiences of that particular shift. When a resident does not feel that any significant new knowledge was added during a shift, the faculty member can respond by helping them to generate a clinical or a scientific question or by asking "what do you *wish* that you knew that would have helped on today's shift?"

Teaching points made during bedside rounds often revolve around the faculty's perception that they are correcting an error made by the resident. Residents often express frustration that they are being taught different things by different faculty members. Although this is an unavoidable part of the residency experience, it is one that encourages residents to make their own judgments. Moreover, it encourages faculty to make corrections in diagnostic or treatment plans in the context of evidence, whenever possible. It is much more credible (and educational) to ask a question about a particular intervention and then answer it together with data from the published literature than to simply insist upon a change in management. Clearly this approach will not always be practical during a busy shift, but a good explanation accompanying such changes is important, and follow-up correspondence with residents is almost always well received. Residents appreciate the special effort that this requires and their learning is enhanced during these interactions.

Lastly, *transcribing* newly assimilated information is a time-honored technique to facilitate neural pathways of memory and improve retention. This can be done in several ways: through written summaries, oral presentations, drawing schematics, or teaching others at the bedside. The most practical and accessible method for residents to integrate lessons from the bedside to their usable fund of knowledge is to keep a written or an electronic journal to record them. These journals can then be edited and revisited throughout the course of the residency – serving as a living, personal textbook to supplement other materials.

## Teaching multitasking

An emergency physician's ability to see multiple patients simultaneously and safely is equally as important as their ability to care for each individual patient. Although formal research into this critical aspect of emergency medical education has only just begun [14–16], many programs have attempted to teach multitasking through the specific structure of their clinical assignments. This usually involves assigning a single resident to a partition or group of beds within the ED for a designated period of time. Structuring assignments in this way brings individual residents' prioritization of time and tasks into focus, in addition to their patient care. We emphasize a two-pass system in the higher acuity areas of the department. In the first assessment, a determination of the acuity of the presentation is made, with time-dependent tasks identified and started. The second assessment focuses on completing the assessment, disposition, and documentation.

## Resident errors

"Primum no nocere" has been a teaching axiom in medicine since the time of Hippocrates, however, errors are a constant reality in medicine. Error rates vary widely in the literature, with estimates of from 3% to 38% of hospitalized patients suffering from an adverse event due to medical error [17]. Error recognition is stressful for residents, but, if managed thoughtfully, errors represent a unique opportunity to facilitate learning [18]. Skillful educators are able to minimize the stress and the negative implications of resident errors while maximizing their educational value – at the bedside, in the conference room, during one-on-one meetings, and in the resident's portfolio.

Learning from resident errors is also an essential part of residency education. Hobgood *et al.* [17] surveyed EM program directors regarding their utilization of resident errors in their programs. Improving performance and changing behavior were the most commonly cited reasons for reporting errors to residents. Less commonly cited reasons included to increase responsibility, enhance compliance, and satisfy requirements of regulatory bodies. Most disclosure of errors occurs during mortality and morbidity conferences, which are a common element of all residencies; however, residents also participate in departmental quality assurance pro-cesses to a variable degree [17]. Residents should participate in the quality assurance process as evaluators as well as evalutees. Being able to evaluate the work of others and possessing an understanding of the peer-review process are minimum prerequisites for leadership roles in community practice.

## Tailoring the individual resident experience

### Systems to improve the continuity of learning

Residents in EM may interact with more than one faculty member during a shift and with many different faculty members during their ED rotations. Moreover, a given resident may not work together with a given faculty member for long intervals of time. It may thus be difficult for some faculty, especially part-time or noncore faculty, to become familiar with each resident's individual strengths and weaknesses. By creating a culture of resident-centeredness and feedback within the residency, residents are more likely to take initiative and responsibility for their own learning agenda.

At our semi-annual "face-to-face" meetings with the residents, we begin with their own self-assessment in each of the core competencies and their progress with the program's written goals and objectives for their level of training. After a review of the objective data and written comments by the faculty (which are organized by core competency) we ask the resident to generate a list of personal objectives for the next six-month period. Specific weaknesses in the core competencies or areas targeted for further excellence are thus identified and formally recorded.

It is widely believed that it is no longer adequate to perform only summative evaluations (e.g. end-of-rotation and semi-annual evaluations) in the absence of real-time feedback during clinical shifts. Most programs use some variation of a direct observation tool or "shift card" as a way to document real-time feedback. To enhance this process, the resident can draw the faculty's attention to their personal objectives at the beginning of a shift. At the end of the shift, the faculty member can then provide feedback that is directed toward the specific weaknesses and needs of the individual resident. Ideally, this feedback is periodically provided to the resident in writing and can become part of the resident's portfolio. These brief reports should be reviewed on an ongoing basis by the residency office faculty and can be used by both the resident and the faculty in the preparation for the next set of personal objectives. They also allow for more timely identification of new problems and adjustment of goals and objectives in the intervals between formal evaluation meetings.

Of course, no real-time feedback mechanism can be successful unless both faculty members and residents feel comfortable giving and receiving it. It is not necessarily natural, nor is it easy to deliver consistently constructive feedback, especially when the performance observed is unacceptable [19]. It may take substantial effort and leadership from the residency office to create a culture where feedback is delivered regularly and thoughtfully by both faculty and residents. It is clear that faculty need feedback to improve as teachers no less than residents require it to improve as learners. Mini-workshops at faculty meetings where experienced teachers give brief examples of effective feedback can stimulate other faculty to improve at this critical skill. Similar workshops are also appropriate for residents, who are also frequent evaluators of junior colleagues and their faculty.

## Remediation

Resident remediation and disciplinary issues can be complex for even the most seasoned program director to navigate. They require knowledge of the relevant legal, institutional, and GME regulations. They also require setting clear expectations of residents in writing, and at the beginning of their training [20]. Although most faculty members will not be responsible for overseeing these issues, their participation in the remediation process cannot be avoided. In *some* cases, it is helpful to have a faculty member external to the residency office act as a coach, mentor, and/or liaison for a resident, because the residency office faculty may be perceived as the ultimate referees of the progress being made. We have utilized this model very successfully in our program. One essential consideration is that the "external" faculty member be agreed upon by all parties.

In most cases, the entire faculty must be aware of and willing to participate in a remediation process. In addition to the residency office keeping the faculty informed at faculty meetings, it is critical for the individual resident to take a leading role by focusing their supervising faculty to their defined areas of weakness.

## Didactic curriculum

Although a discussion of an EM residency didactic curriculum is not the focus of this chapter, the effect of the didactic program on the clinical teaching program is important. In contrast to most medical and surgical training programs, it is difficult to link the didactic and the clinical portions of the curriculum together. Residents in the ED see undifferentiated patients of all demographic groups from their first day forward, regardless of what topics they have covered in their conferences and readings. At our program, which uses a module-based system to cover the essential knowledge base of the specialty, we have recently modified the curriculum to ensure that all of the most frequently encountered patient presentations are dealt with early in the schedule. We have also introduced a greater deal of redundancy in the curriculum, by formally repeating core topics such as electrocardiography, pediatric fever evaluation, and neurological emergencies in each year level, while introducing progressively more advanced concepts and literature at each stage. It is also clearly beneficial to engage the faculty at large in this process, with the curriculum readily available to them so that they may use it as a framework to gauge the residents' knowledge base and be acquainted with their learning materials. Making as much of the curricular material available online through a group server is an excellent way to accomplish this.

### Summary

Clinical teaching in an EM residency should never be taken for granted. Over time, relationships between individual faculty members and residents evolve, enabling teaching and supervisory activities to be tailored to resident-specific educational goals. Although it is our hope that some of the background and suggestions that we have offered in this discussion are helpful, they can only serve as a starting point for motivated faculty. Ultimately, the best clinical teachers improve only by listening carefully and responding to the feedback of their two main constituent groups: the residents and their patients.

# References

1. Beeson M, Gerson L, Weigand J, Jwayyed S, Kuhn G. Characteristics of emergency medicine program directors. *Acad Emerg Med* 2006; 13(2): 166–172.

2. Whitehead D, Thomas HJ, Slapper D. A rational approach to shift work in emergency medicine. *Ann Emerg Med* 1992; 21(10): 1250–1258.

3. Smith-Coggins R, Rosekind M, Buccino K, Dinges D, Moser R. Rotating shiftwork schedules: can we enhance physician adaptation to night shifts? *Acad Emerg Med* 1997; 4(10): 951–961.

4. Chisholm C, Whenmouth L, Daly E, Cordell W, Giles B, Brizendine E. An evaluation of emergency medicine resident interaction time with

faculty in different teaching venues. *Acad Emerg Med* 2004; 11(2): 149–155.

5. Shayne P, Heilpern K, Ander D, Palmer-Smith V. Protected clinical teaching time and a bedside clinical evaluation instrument in an emergency medicine training program. *Acad Emerg Med* 2002; 9(11): 1342–1349.

6. Stahmer S, Ellison S, Jubanyik K, *et al.* Integrating the core competencies: proceedings from the 2005 Academic Assembly consortium. *Acad Emerg Med* 2007; 14(1): 80–94.

7. Dyne P, Strauss R, Rinnert S. Systems-based practice: the sixth core competency. *Acad Emerg Med* 2002; 9(11): 1270–1277.

8. Bandiera G, Lee S, Tiberius R. Creating effective learning in today's emergency departments: how accomplished teachers get it done. *Ann Emerg Med* 2005; 45(3): 253–261.

9. Thurgur L, Bandiera G, Lee S, Tiberius R. What do emergency medicine learners want from their teachers? A multicenter focus group analysis. *Acad Emerg Med* 2005; 12(9): 856–861.

10. Atzema C, Bandiera G, Schull M. Emergency department crowding: the effect on resident education. *Ann Emerg Med* 2005; 45(3): 276–281.

11. Penciner R. Clinical teaching in a busy emergency department: strategies for success. *CJEM* 2002; 4(4): 286–288.

12. Silverman ME, Murray TJ, Bryan CS (eds). *The Quotable Osler*. American College of Physicians, Philadelphia, 2003.

13. Ellis D, Lerner E, Jehle D, Romano K, Siffring C. A multi-state survey of videotaping practices for major trauma resuscitations. *J Emerg Med* 1999; 17(4): 597–604.

14. Chisholm C, Collison E, Nelson D, Cordell W. Emergency department workplace interruptions: are emergency physicians "interrupt-driven" and "multitasking"? *Acad Emerg Med* 2000; 7(11): 1239–1243.

15. Laxmisan A, Hakimzada F, Sayan O, Green R, Zhang J, Patel V. The multitasking clinician: decision-making and cognitive demand during and after team handoffs in emergency care. *Int J Med Inform* 2007; 76(11–12): 801–811.

16. Kobayashi L, Shapiro M, Gutman D, Jay G. Multiple encounter simulation for high-acuity multipatient environment training. *Acad Emerg Med* 2007; 14(12): 1141–1148.

17. Hobgood C, Ma O, Swart G. Emergency medicine resident errors: identification and educational utilization. *Acad Emerg Med* 2000; 7(11): 1317–1320.

18. Wu A, Folkman S, McPhee S, Lo B. Do house officers learn from their mistakes? *JAMA* 1991; 265(16): 2089–2094.

19. Dudek N, Marks M, Regehr G. Failure to fail: the perspectives of clinical supervisors. *Acad Med* 2005; 80(10 Suppl): S84–S87.

20. Smith C, Stevens N, Servis M. A general framework for approaching residents in difficulty. *Fam Med* 2007; 39(5): 331–336.

# CHAPTER 12

# Teaching physicians in training how to teach

*Carey D. Chisholm*
*Indiana University School of Medicine, Indianapolis, IN, USA*

## Teaching residents how to teach

When a resident (U.S. term for a post-graduate physician in a specialty training program) enters their training program, there is no mandate that they possess good teaching skills. Nevertheless, residents assume teaching responsibilities almost immediately. The ACGME (Accreditation Council for Graduate Medical Education – the U.S. oversight body that sets post-graduate training requirements) recognizes the value of the teaching role of residents, and incorporates that requirement as part of the training accreditation process [1, 2]. Due to training proximity, residents often possess insight about learner needs and knowledge deficiencies. In addition, learners are often more relaxed and forthcoming since residents occupy "lower tiers" in the academic hierarchy. The "teaching skill set" that residents must develop does not differ dramatically from that of faculty (Table 12.1). This chapter focuses on non-procedural clinical teaching in the emergency department (ED) itself. Since the emergency medicine (EM) resident most frequently interfaces with fourth year (senior level) medical students (MS4), this chapter focuses on that interaction.

The unique ED practice environment creates many challenges for the resident teacher [3, 4]. The initial challenge is developing accurate and realistic expectations of the learner capabilities. Table 12.2 lists several additional challenges facing the EM resident.

## Setting teaching expectations

Recognize the anxiety accompanying the majority of MS4s as they begin their rotations in our complex EDs. Before jumping right to

*Practical Teaching in Emergency Medicine*, 1st edition. Edited by R Rogers, A Mattu, M Winters & J Martinez. ©2009 Blackwell Publishing, ISBN: 9781405176224

**Table 12.1** The resident "teaching skill set".

---

- Didactic presentations
  - Grand rounds and lectures
  - Less structured (e.g. case conference)
  - Small groups and workshops
- Clinical venue
  - Procedures
  - Bedside
  - Away from the bedside
- Learner assessment
- Written educational materials

---

**Table 12.2** Challenges of teaching in the Emergency Department.

---

- Understanding/assessing learner needs
- Learner inexperience:
  - With acute disease presentations
  - Gaps in knowledge base
  - Limited experience with cultural and social issues
  - Transitioning from information gatherer to assimilator
- Balancing individual patient care needs with education activities
- Balancing overall patient flow with teaching multiple learners
- Adapting and adjusting to a "flexible" teaching style
- Appropriate use and access of educational resources (articles, web, and so on)
- Assessing learner performance

---

patient care, it is helpful to defuse some of their anxiety. It is important to set the "educational stage". Consider starting the shift by asking some of the questions listed in Table 12.3. This places the learner at greater ease, and sets the tone and expectations for your time together.

Senior students have large gaps in their experiential and cognitive database. Often the MS4 has never encountered or cared for a patient with the chief complaint, signs, or symptoms now confronting them. Conversely, their general knowledge base may appear artificially strong if they have had a recent in-depth clinical experience with similar patients (e.g. their familiarity with doing a slit lamp examination immediately following an Ophthalmology rotation). The following questions are helpful in developing realistic expectations of your learner:

- Have you ever taken care of a patient with this illness before?
- Are you comfortable doing this portion of the physical examination?

**Table 12.3** Getting to know the learner.

- Where did you grow up?
- Where did you go to undergraduate school?
- What is your medical school/specialty choice?
- Have you worked in the ED before?
- What would you like to learn more about during this shift?
- Do you understand that it is fine to say "I don't know", but I am relying on you to be completely honest in your answers to me today?

If the response to either of the initial questions is "no", ask them accompany you as you model the approach to the patient. This often saves the patient, the student, and you a large amount of frustration.

> CAVEAT: Explain to the learner that the *only* way to get into trouble is to delay care for a sick patient. Assure that they understand that you want them to alert you at any time they encounter somebody who appears to be significantly ill.

The majority of MS4s have little experience in critical thinking about patients. Prior rotations largely reinforce the role of "data gatherer" with the more senior team members doing the "data synthesis" components. Because their prior clinical training on inpatient services reinforced and rewarded thoroughness of data gathering, one can anticipate that this component is overdone. The EM rotation is designed to teach them the "broad strokes" of caring for patients with a wide array of undifferentiated conditions. Questions useful in teaching these "broad strokes" are listed in Table 12.4.

Do not underestimate the difficulty that these seemingly simplistic ideas may pose to your novice learner . Using these questions decreases the likelihood of encountering the robotic "inpatient presentation" style of regurgitating unfiltered historical data. Note these questions are specific and directive. Your learner will quickly ascertain that critical thinking and focus are the expectation during their ED rotation.

> CAVEAT: request that all presentations start with a review of any abnormalities of the vital signs at some point during the first 15 seconds of discussion.

**Table 12.4** Helpful questions used to teach the "broad strokes" of emergency care.

---

- Is this patient "sick" or "not sick"?
- What do you think the most likely diagnosis is?
- Do you think this patient will be able to go home, go home with close follow-up within 1–2 days, or require admission to the hospital?
- If you could only order one test for this patient, what would it be?
- Tell me three things that could kill/harm this patient if not diagnosed today?

---

In general, discussions should assure a focus on the "ED approach" to a symptom complex or chief complaint. This includes an emphasis on teaching the ED "rule out the worst case scenario" approach to symptom complexes. Diagramming your thought process as you discuss the case provides an additional visual learning tool, and is particularly helpful in these general "approach to" scenarios. However, flexibility and situational awareness of your work environment is critical, lest patients inadvertently be inconvenienced or even harmed. During high volume periods it is appropriate to become directive and specific [5, 7]. The role flexes from teacher to supervisor. In these situations, encouraging your learner to jot down their questions for later discussion affords the opportunity to close the loop, and reinforce important concepts. For instance, "Why do you think I asked you to order that head CAT scan so quickly for the patient with the sudden onset of the worst headache of their life" or "Why did we order steroids for the teenager with the wheezing"? It is common to have multiple learners simultaneously. This may create a queue of learners waiting to staff their cases. Just as we triage patients according to acuity, quickly explore which patient may be most important to see next by asking, "Who has a patient that requires admission?" or "Who has a patient with abnormal vital signs?"

The ED patient population is replete with "difficult" or "challenging" patients. MS4s have rarely encountered this spectrum of humanity with the accompanying complex psychosocial issues. They can easily become frustrated about caring for such patients. Teach your learner questions that can help them provide appropriate care for the difficult patient. A sample of questions to ask such patients is listed in Table 12.5.

"Finalizing" a patient encounter affords an excellent opportunity to assure the proper care plan is instituted. This also provides you the chance to ensure that the learner has assimilated the major

**Table 12.5** Helpful questions when caring for a "difficult" ED patient.

---

- What do you think is causing you to feel this way?
- What are you hoping that we can accomplish for you here in the ED today?
- When symptoms have been present for more than several days: "What changed to make you decide to come in now as opposed to 12 hours ago or 2–3 days ago"?
- If I could only fix one of your problems, which one would you want me to fix?
- Are you supposed to take any medications each day for any health problem?
- Have you started taking any new medicines, changed the dose of any medicines, or stopped taking any medicines in the past 5 days?
- Have you ever been in the hospital overnight as a patient?

---

**Table 12.6** Useful questions for "finalizing" an ED patient visit.

---

- What does the patient need to understand regarding their follow-up?
- What did you find most challenging about this patient?
- What would you do differently the next time you care for a similar patient?
- What's the most important thing to remember when caring for a future similar patient?

---

points you taught them. Questions useful for finalizing the patient encounter are listed in Table 12.6.

Although there are many challenges to teaching in the ED, there are likewise many opportunities to engage in creative teaching activities, particularly in areas of predictable learner inexperience. A sample of these activities is listed in Table 12.7.

## Pitfalls of resident teaching

Resident teachers will invariably face challenges and potential pitfalls. The major pitfalls encountered by resident teachers are listed in Table 12.8.

Balancing creative techniques with the predictable pitfalls of teaching is a learned skill requiring practice and ongoing effort [5]. Do not equate ED systems knowledge with clinical knowledge and capabilities. The longer one works in the same ED, the more removed one becomes from feeling these pressures. Our teaching EDs are extremely complex, with multiple layers of potential confusion ranging from patient assignment, ordering treatment or tests, accessing data, and discharging the patient. Residents often can more easily recall the systems issues that plagued their early

**Table 12.7** Teaching techniques.

- Act the part of the consultant on the phone prior to placing the call
- Act the part of the family member inquiring about the treatment plan
- Act the part of the patient who will receive bad news
- "Dry run" the procedure step by step on a colleague
- Scripted 1–2 minutes discussions about common diseases
- Pre-selected web sites, text tables, articles, photos
- Teaching files of "classic" EKGs
- Draw and outline key components

**Table 12.8** Pitfalls in resident teaching.

- Assuming the learner can navigate the ED system
- Teaching too much about a given patient (focus on 2–3 "take home" points)
- Focusing on what interests them, as opposed to what the learner needs to know
- Teaching specifics rather than concepts
- Teaching concepts when directive specifics are necessary
- Usurping care without explaining why
- Failing to be directive when patient care is potentially compromised
- Answering one's own question
- Failure to explain the difference between personal treatment preference and evidence-based treatment
- Correcting/counseling/reprimanding where others can overhear

shifts. Anticipate that your learner will have difficulty maneuvering through the system. Remember, they are there to learn the "broad strokes" of our specialty, not the intimate quirks and nuances of your ED. It is even more helpful if you anticipate system roadblocks and intervene accordingly.

The second common pitfall stems from the tendency of the teacher to emphasize things that are of personal interest and confidence, rather than items of learner need. Paradoxically, the more "expertise" you have in a subject area, the more likely you are to stray here. For instance, rather than discussing the fundamental components of wound care, you instead focus on rarely encountered complicating situations (e.g. wound botulism). The learner often has difficulty prioritizing such information, and may erroneously generalize the exception into the norm.

Attempting to teach "too much" about each case is a major pitfall for early clinical teachers. It simply seems appropriate to try to share everything one knows about the management of a disease process with the learner. Do not attempt to cover "too much" information with the learner. Rather than a comprehensive discussion about the ED management of asthma, envision what you would wish your learner to be able to recall about the topic 6 months from now. Focus your teaching on these 2–3 points. More than three invariably will lessen recall or inadvertently create improper emphasis. By developing "scripted" 1–2 minute overview synopses about common complaints such as pharyngitis or back pain, you communicate key information efficiently. Use electronic files or paper copies of important material to reinforce your message. Examples include "The rational clinical examination. Does this patient have strep throat?" [6], Ottawa Ankle Rules, or physical therapy exercises diagram for low back pain. Electronic databases afford rapid access to clinical images, radiographs, and EKGs to augment the teaching interaction. Keep a list of helpful sites easily accessible and consciously include them in your teaching process.

It is also tempting to teach about topics you are most familiar and comfortable with. Try to maintain a perspective about the needs of your learner as opposed to your desires and interests about teaching content. This is particularly true as you develop "expertise" about a subject and your natural enthusiasm will push you towards sharing subtle nuances as opposed to the more needed generalization.

Just as there are difficult patients, there will be challenging learners. Avoidance of certain chief complaints is common, and stems from fear of the unknown (learner does not know how to even start the case) to poor work effort. Conversely, some learners are so enthused that they quickly may assume care for too many patients. In both situations you must become more directive, either dealing out patients from the pick-up list, or asking the overextended learner to check in before assuming a new case. Physicians already in training may display variable interest in patient populations they will likely not encounter in the future, such as the internal medicine resident avoiding the febrile infant. Be creative in finding ways to make such cases more interesting to the learner ("What is this was your child/grandparent/family asking advice?").

It is awkward to wait for a learner to answer a question. At times this stems from the obtuse nature of the query, leaving the learner playing the "Guess what I'm thinking" game. In general, give the learner time … up to 15 seconds … to develop a response. If the learner struggles, consider rephrasing the question, or alternatively gaining closure by stating, "OK, go ahead and give me your best guess".

Anticipate the learner's inexperience in dealing with phone consultants and with sensitive patient–family communications. Do not set them up to fail, particularly when you expect potentially difficult interactions (the "crusty" consultant or breaking the news of a probable lung cancer found on CAT scan). By "play-acting" the role of the consultant or patient beforehand, you build confidence in your learner and may effectively steer them away from trouble. Stand nearby to monitor the consultant conversation, and in the situation of delivering bad news, you may wish to model this technique for the learner, or at lest accompany them to the patient's room.

There are several behaviors universally resented by learners. The first is usurping care from them without providing an explanation about why you did so. Tactfully but truthfully providing this information is important to learner development. The second is failure to explain the difference between one's personal management preferences, and those firmly established in evidence-based practice. Much of ED practice lacks the scientific support of large well-designed randomized controlled trials. Communication about clear evidence as opposed to personal preference in the absence of such is important. Criticizing the learner in the presence of others, particularly patients, families or their peers, creates resentment and impedes learning. The ED physical plant challenges the recommendation to "praise in public, perfect in private". One must be particularly tactful and aware at the bedside. Develop scripted replies for use when your learner struggles such as "That's a very interesting thought" or "That approach works nicely for many patients, but in this situation I think we will use this alternative".

## Learner assessment

Closing the loop by providing formal feedback to the learner is an important component of the clinical teaching process [7–9]. In developing feedback, it is useful to break the patient encounter into three discrete "compartments": data gathering, data synthesis, and communication/professionalism. Assign a "grade" (e.g. Honors, High Pass, Pass, and so on) to each individual compartment, then combine for a composite "patient grade". Using the "patient grades", one develops a composite shift grade. The information gathering aspect analyzes the history, physical examination and use of ancillary information (family, emergency medical service (EMS) records, nursing notes, and so on). The data synthesis component examines the therapeutic plan (diagnostic tests, treatments, disposition, involvement of consultants, and so on).

Communication/professionalism items include starting the shift on time, attire, work ethic, presentation skills, charting, interactions with consultants, nursing/prehospital care providers and secretaries, and bedside discussions with the patient and family. Note that you cannot accurately assess much of the data gathering and the majority of the communication/professionalism components without conducting direct observation of the learner. Whenever possible, conduct these observations without alerting the learner, for humans tend to change their behavior when they know they are being watched. You may do this by serptiously standing just outside the exam room door or behind the curtain and listening to the conversation, or near the student as they speak with a consultant on the phone.

## Staying organized as a teacher

Although it may at times be difficult to manage your own patient load during a busy ED shift, the complexity seemingly increases logarithmically when sheparding multiple learners through the care of their patients. It behooves you to develop a method to organize the care process for patients under your supervisory responsibility. How and what information you record is less important than assuring the method works for you. At minimum, capture the patient's age and sex, location, presenting complaint, and components of their management plan. You may also wish to have a code to annotate after you have evaluated the patient yourself, informed your faculty about the patient, and written a note on the medical record. Use this form to also capture specific observations that you wish to incorporate into your summative evaluation of the shift. For instance, "understood empiric therapy for Strep throat, including CENTOR" or "explained treatment plan without using medical jargon". These take seconds to record during the shift, but provide the details to allow more than platitudes such as "good job" that learners find to be of minimum benefit.

## Conclusion

The recommendations presented in this chapter are a compilation of teaching techniques of use in "ideal" circumstances. It is uncommon to bring all of these into play on even a single patient encounter. Instead, the resident teacher must experiment with using varying components as time and patient flow permit. Setting a goal to incorporate several of these over the course of a shift is realistic, and greatly appreciated by the learner. Learners appreciate enthusiastic, receptive, and interested teachers. They have significant gaps in their knowledge base and clinical skills, and this coupled with the demands of real-time ED patient flow mandate a flexible approach to teaching. Conceptually, dividing the patient encounter into information acquisition, data synthesis, and communication/professionalism permits a more realistic performance expectation and assessment. Direct observation of the learner permits evaluation of aspects of data gathering and communication/professionalism otherwise not readily assessed. By anticipating system pitfalls and navigating the student through those, the resident teacher more effectively balances patient and learner needs. It is important to develop an organizational tool to allow tracking of patient progress and performance specifics of merit to incorporate into a summative evaluation.

## Summary points

- Set expectations for the learner
- Be an enthusiastic and approachable teacher
- Anticipate problems with navigating the ED system
- Anticipate significant knowledge/clinical experiential gaps
- Review patient vital signs early in the encounter
- Model novel patient care situations for the learner
- Conceptually break the patient encounter into information gathering, data synthesis, and communication/professionalism components
- Do not try to teach too many concepts for any given patient
- Develop "scripted" educational sound bites and questions for your learners
- Play-act the role of a consultant, patient or family to "dry run" a difficult communication
- Be flexible in the use of time and teaching style depending upon ambient ED conditions
- Develop a system to monitor the progress of your learners' patients
- "Finalize" patient encounters with the learner

**Tips for EM educators supervizing resident teaching efforts in the ED**

- Directly observe the teaching activity, and provide feedback
- Do not usurp a teaching encounter unless the resident is clearly floundering
- Model novel educational situations
- Share your organizational techniques for monitoring patient care
- Share informational databases you use as educational adjuncts
- Ask what they hope the learner will recall about caring for a patient with a similar clinical condition in the future
- Play-act the role of the learner for a given situation
- Challenge the resident to look for "non-medical" teaching opportunities during patient encounters (ethics, professional, societal)
- Do not discredit the resident in front of the learner (have tactful methods to move the encounter along, then share your concerns privately)

# References

1. ACGME (Accreditation Council for Graduate Medical Education), *Common Program Requirements*. 2007.
2. Farrell SE, *et al.*, Resident-as-teacher: A suggested curriculum for emergency medicine. *Acad Emerg Med* 2006; 13(6): 677–679.
3. Chisholm CD, *et al.*, Emergency department workplace interruptions: Are emergency physicians "interrupt-driven" and "multitasking"? [see comment]. *Acad Emerg Med* 2000; 7(11): 1239–1243.
4. Chisholm CD, *et al.*, Work interrupted: a comparison of workplace interruptions in emergency departments and primary care offices. *Ann Emerg Med* 2001; 38(2): 146–151.
5. Bandiera G, Lee S, Tiberius R, Creating effective learning in today's emergency departments: How accomplished teachers get it done. *Ann Emerg Med* 2005; 45(3): 253–261.
6. Ebell MH, *et al.*, The rational clinical examination. Does this patient have strep throat? *JAMA* 2000; 284(22): 2912–2918.
7. Thurgur L, *et al.*, What do emergency medicine learners want from their teachers? A multicenter focus group analysis. *Acad Emerg Med* 2005; 12(9): 856–861.
8. Torre DM, Sebastian JL, Simpson DE, Learning activities and high-quality teaching: perceptions of third-year IM clerkship students. *Acad Med* 2003; 78(8): 812–814.
9. Torre DM, *et al.*, Learning/feedback activities and high-quality teaching: perceptions of third-year medical students during an inpatient rotation. *Acad Med* 2005; 80(10): 950–954.

# Improving as an Educator in Emergency Medicine

# CHAPTER 13

# Characteristics of great teachers

*Jennifer Avegno[1], Peter M. C. DeBlieux[2]*
[1]*Medical Student Clerkship Director, LSUHSC Section of Emergency Medicine, New Orleans, LA, USA*
[2]*Director of Resident & Faculty Development, Section of Emergency Medicine, Professor of Clinical Medicine, Staff Physician, Pulmonary/Critical Care, New Orleans, LA, USA*

As Emergency Medicine (EM) has developed and become a formal specialty, attention to its unique learning environment and methods of educating trainees has increased. Gone are the days of "see one – do one – teach one" in the Emergency Department (ED); as with other medical specialties, the value of refining, standardizing, and devoting study to specific educational practices has become increasingly important. Formal and informal teaching has been studied and described in other medical settings – the hospital ward, the outpatient clinic – the ED presents distinct opportunities and challenges to both teaching and learning.

In the ED, there is a higher degree of interruption than a clinic or hospital ward, and learning opportunities are available around the clock, rather than just during normal business hours. EM educators must address the needs of student and resident rotators from a wide variety of specialties, rather than a monospecialty team. Shift times may be asynchronous among levels of training, leading to "no good time" for dedicated learning. Institutional pressure for patient flow and efficiency is often at odds with the desire for dedicated educational time. Learners and educators must be aware of these constraints while recognizing that the ED provides the best exposure to undifferentiated patient cases and the ability to follow a case from inception to diagnosis to treatment and disposition.

What makes a great teacher in the special environment of the ED? Some EM-specific research highlights widely accepted characteristics of

*Practical Teaching in Emergency Medicine*, 1st edition. Edited by R Rogers, A Mattu, M Winters & J Martinez. ©2009 Blackwell Publishing, ISBN: 9781405176224

superior educators, and is in agreement with evidence presented from other medical specialties. In order to fully understand what makes an EM teacher great, one must explore what learners themselves want from their teachers and what established EM teachers consider good practice. Also important is the consideration of different teaching styles in the unique ED setting and identifying barriers to great teaching.

## What do learners want from their teachers?

Several studies based in ambulatory clinics or hospital wards have identified what learners – medical students and residents – believe are characteristics of good teachers. A meta-analysis of the characteristics of effective clinical teachers and their teaching methods revealed that educators take on several important roles: an effective supervisor, a dynamic teacher, a role model, and a supportive person [1]. These roles shift in preference depending on the learner's level – medical students generally prefer the traditional instructional role when the teacher controls the environment, whereas residents more frequently describe good teachers as those who are supervisors and supportive of their autonomy [2].

From each specific educational experience, learners value teachers with enthusiasm, clearly stated answers and objectives, opportunities for problem-solving, and a true mentoring relationship with their educators [3]. A focus group of internal medicine residents identified a set of characteristics for "skilled" bedside teachers – arguably the most frequent type of instruction readily available in an ED. They concluded that faculty who had the ability to conduct timely, efficient, and beneficial bedside instruction for a variety of learner levels, and were unafraid of the barriers to bedside teaching, had the greatest success in this particular medical setting [4].

Studies of EM learners mirror the above findings. A focus group of students, residents, and off-service intern ED rotators developed several consensus principles of effective teachers: those who seize the teachable moment, give appropriate feedback, are learner-centered, have a good attitude, and are good role models with effective teaching skills [5]. The teacher's level of training (resident, junior or senior staff) was found to be unimportant if teaching was tailored to the learner's needs. Other educator characteristics that EM learners value include efficiency, organization, knowledge base, adaptability to barriers, and respect for patients [6].

Synthesis of the above research on both EM and non-EM based learner preferences reveals several core truths (see Box 13.1).

> **Box 13.1** What do learners think makes a great teacher?
>
> "Seize the moment"
> Learner-centered
> Professional role model
> Enthusiasm
> Overcomes educational barriers
> Efficient and organized
> Strong knowledge base

Perhaps most appropriate to the ED, educators who take time to teach – or "seize the teachable moment" – without fear of the many barriers to instruction are highly valued by learners. Enthusiastic role models who are learner-centered in their approach deliver the highest quality educational experience. This places demands on the educator – how to tailor instruction to a wide variety of learner backgrounds and styles? – but the best teachers are able to provide this in an efficient, organized manner.

## What do medical educators believe are characteristics of great teachers?

Although learner preferences are important, historically medical education has progressed "on the shoulders of giants" (i.e. with each generation of excellent teachers learning from those preceding it). Only in recent times has serious study been given to investigate *why* great teachers were considered great, and how they imparted their knowledge and methods to their students. With the premise that all teachers are learners first, several studies of accomplished physician educators have investigated how these instructors achieved success. The influence of positive role models was unanimously stated, particularly important since many teachers receive little or no formal educational training or supervision [7, 8]. Even fewer physician educators receive focused training in educational principles that facilitate their roles. Institutional encouragement, recognition and promotion of formal and informal teaching, and establishing dedicated time strictly for education, was also seen as critical for the development of excellent medical educators.

Other educators across specialties have proposed characteristics of the "ideal" medical teacher – stimulating, encouraging, competent,

**Box 13.2** What do great teachers think leads to their success?

Positive role model
Learner-centered
Positive attitude/enthusiasm
Adaptability
Patient care and involvement
Ability to "seize the moment"

communicative, and knowledgeable [9]. An expert opinion described habits of effective clinical teachers, namely: focusing on learner needs, thinking out loud (i.e. making clear the reasoning behind decisions or statements), remaining clear and simple, linking learning to patient care and kindness, adapting and embracing any situation, and demonstrating good listening skills [10]. These habits were reiterated in a survey of teachers and students in the ambulatory setting, where involving and stimulating learners, and offering clear expectations with skillful patient care significantly predicted overall teaching effectiveness [11].

In a survey of accomplished (award-winning or highly promoted) EM teachers, several strategies were identified that contributed to a superior learning experience. In short, these educators believed that all of the following contributed to their own educational success: learner-centered activity, tailoring teaching to the situation and environment, acting as a role model with a good attitude, and efficient use of all available resources [12]. Teachers who focus their information on the needs and levels of the learner, in an environment where expectations are clear and mutually agreeable, and show active involvement in patient care have the greatest success. These educators also suggest that having different teaching strategies on hand for any situation – busy or slow times, day or night, with solitary students or with a mixed group of learners – allows them to deliver a consistent product regardless of circumstance.

Teachers of medicine tend to agree with learners on their ideal characteristics for an educator (see Box 13.2). Primarily, educators should be learner-centered – focusing on the learner's needs, demonstrate a competent level of training, engaged in patient care, and able to target specific objectives in the educational exercise. Teachers are also expected to *"carpe diem"* – seize any learning opportunity that arises without regard to institutional, environmental, or time pressures that exist. Efficiency, organization, and preparation are crucial for success. Perhaps the most important – but also least tangible – requirement for great teachers is that they act as positive, enthusiastic role models with an excellent attitude. These approaches maintain the time-honored tradition of mentoring medical professionals as an important function in modern education.

## What styles do great teachers use?

There are several general lecture styles that teachers may use to convey information. The oldest and most common style in medical education is the didactic lecture. In this format, the teacher conveys his/her knowledge unidirectionally to a group of learners with little interruption for questions or interactive discourse. While this is a common and efficient strategy utilized in medical education due to the sheer volume of knowledge and poor student–teacher ratios, it may be inefficient and not ideal for standard on-shift teaching in a busy ED [13].

An interactive style of teaching, with a steady flow of questions and answers between teacher and learner, is more engaging and often more appropriate for the ED. Superior educators are skilled at maximizing the yield from a series of focused questions in order to stimulate learning. These teachers ask clear, targeted questions appropriate to the learners' levels, allow for multiple correct responses, use queries that require more sophisticated thought than a simple yes/no, and – perhaps most importantly – allow sufficient wait times (3 seconds or more) for a response [8, 13].

In addition to strict lecture and questioning styles, EM teachers may have opportunity to provide direct demonstration of a particular technique or procedure to students and residents. This may be somewhat time-consuming and inefficient, but quite effective in providing proper training in a skill set that is perhaps infrequently seen or performed in the ED. This demonstrative style can ultimately foster learner autonomy as it provides them with a standard skill set that they can then work to achieve.

A simple "microskills" model of clinical teaching has been proposed that provides a framework for structuring the educational experience [14]. The first two tenets of this model are learner-centered: "get a commitment" (allow the learner to present and commit to solving

> **Box 13.3** The "microskills" model of clinical teaching
>
> Get a commitment
> Probe for supporting evidence
> Teach general rules
> Reinforce what's right
> Correct mistakes

a particular case or problem) and "probe for evidence" (by analyzing the learner's reasoning, gaps in their knowledge or thought process can be ascertained). The educator then teaches "general rules" – standardized bits of knowledge targeted to the learner's level. Finally, the teacher "reinforces what's right" – supporting accurate knowledge – and "corrects mistakes" by discussing errors and how to prevent them in the future. These last three microskills are geared towards tailoring teaching to the learner and building a foundation for future knowledge. By remaining learner-centered, this model gives learners what they seek and allows great teachers to deliver a consistent experience.

Choosing a unique educational style – but remaining flexible within the constraints of each situation – is another hallmark of a successful educator. Having a set of well-rehearsed "teaching scripts" on hand that can be applied to a variety of cases is a popular strategy among clinical teachers [3, 15]. Great educators choose their teaching cases wisely, and focus on those that will maximize learning broad concepts. Teachers must also be flexible in their personal style – alternatively authoritative, collaborative, suggestive, or collegial – where appropriate to the situation. In the constantly changing environment of the ED, great teachers marry a set of tried-and-true teaching styles with the current needs of the learner group and demands of the circumstances at hand.

## What are environmental adjuncts and barriers to successful teachers?

Numerous barriers to teaching effectively have been detailed, both by medical educators and learners and may be divided into learner, teacher, and environmental obstacles [4, 10, 12]. Learner barriers include a lack of interest, preparation, time, and resources. Teacher-centered impediments include frequent lack of time and available resources, discouragement of teaching in favor of billable activities or research, mastery of patient case detail, lack of formal teaching skills, and personal factors such as burnout and ego. Environmental obstacles include the physical makeup of the physical setting, variability in patient cases, and overall support for teaching within the institution. EM teachers face additional challenges not seen by the ward or clinic; there is often no prior relationship with the patient, and their condition or diagnosis is often unknown at the time of interaction (i.e. the undifferentiated sick patient), and the high degree of interruption facing every busy ED.

As noted above, successful teachers are undaunted by the many challenges to medical education. Indeed, available evidence shows that environmental or workload constraints have no significant effect on teaching scores [6, 11]. Learners ranked those teachers highest who had excellent teaching skills, showed willingness to teach, and established a positive learning environment – irrespective of the available patient case mix, faculty workload, or design of the clinical site.

Great teachers use what is available to them. They are aware of the unique obstacles to high-quality education in the modern, busy ED but develop strategies to minimize these impediments. Using the microskills model, some have proposed a "one-minute teaching" strategy – learners and teacher perform a history and physical exam together, then learners commit to a diagnosis while the teacher assesses reasoning and focuses on a *single* teaching point, corrects mistakes, and reinforces correct thinking [3]. Even a busy ED shift is permeated with multiple "one-minute" opportunities for the successful teacher to identify.

In the ED, great educators know patient flow well enough to identify traditionally less busy times where dedicated teaching might occur, and may utilize unused areas within the department – a code area that is kept open but rarely occupied, for instance – for fewer interruptions during instruction. Other creative solutions include regular, weekly "board rounds" – both on and off-shift faculty, residents, and students meet for a brief period in the ED to discuss and teach about currently active cases. This provides for fresh perspective, positively impacts patient care, and uses available resources for problem solving [16].

## Conclusion

Great teachers of EM are a diverse group of clinicians and academicians, but the core behaviors and principles that promote their success are standard. A primary focus on learners, enthusiasm

and proper role modeling, adaptability and an undaunted ability
to seize the teachable moment are all as important as a strong
knowledge base and clinical acumen. What learners and teachers
want is the same: to provide the best possible educational experience
in any available setting. Though the ED is a unique environment
with its own special challenges, good teachers employ simple but
powerful strategies for success.

---

### Summary points

- The ED is a learning and teaching environment like no other, and
  educators must be aware of the unique advantages and constraints
  to imparting information.
- EM learners value teachers who "seize the moment," are
  enthusiastic, and adaptive to a variety of learner backgrounds and
  styles.
- Great EM educators should be learner-centered, well-trained,
  directly engaged in patient care, efficient and organized, and
  aware of their status as role models.
- Various teaching styles may be employed by EM educators,
  including a microskills model, teaching scripts, and using single
  cases to illustrate broad concepts.
- Though significant time and resource-related barriers exist to
  effective teaching in the ED, successful educators use what is available
  to them and develop strategies to minimize these challenges.

---

## References

1. Irby DM. Teaching and learning in ambulatory care settings: A thematic review of the literature. *Acad Med* 1995; 70: 898–931.
2. Paukert JL, Richards BF. How medical students and residents describe the roles and characteristics of their influential clinical teachers. *Acad Med* 75: 843–845.
3. Parsell G, Bligh J. Recent perspectives on clinical teaching. *Med Educ* 2001; 35: 409–414.
4. Ramani S, Orlander JD, Strunin L, Barber TW. Whither bedside teaching? A focus-group study of clinical teachers. *Acad Med* 2003; 78: 384–390.
5. Thurgur L, Bandiera G, Lee S, Tiberius R. What do emergency medicine learners want from their teachers? A multicenter focus group analysis. *Acad Emerg Med* 2005; 12: 856–861.

6. Kelly SP, Shapiro N, Woodruff M, Corrigan K, Sanchez LD, Wolfe RE. The effects of clinical workload on teaching in the emergency department. *Acad Emerg Med* 2007; 526–531.
7. MacDougall J, Drummond MJ. The development of medical teachers: An enquiry into the learning histories of 10 experienced medical teachers. *Med Educ* 2005; 39: 1213–1220.
8. Hekelman FP, Blase JR. Excellence in clinical teaching: the core of the mission. *Acad Med* 1996; 71: 738–742.
9. Morrison EH, Hitchcock MA, Harthill M, Boker JR, Masunaga H. The on-line clinical teaching perception inventory: A "snapshot" of medical teachers. *Fam Med* 2005; 37: 48–53.
10. Reilly BM. Inconvenient truths about effective clinical teaching. *Lancet* 2007; 370: 705–711.
11. Irby DM, Ramsey PG, Gillmore GM, Schaad D. Characteristics of effective clinical teachers of ambulatory care medicine. *Acad Med* 1991; 66: 54–55.
12. Bandiera G, Lee S, Tiberius R. Creating effective learning in today's emergency departments: How accomplished teachers get it done. *Ann Emerg Med* 2005; 45: 253–261.
13. Penciner R. Clinical teaching in a busy emergency department: Strategies for success. *Can J Emerg Med* 2002; 4: 286–288.
14. Neber JO, Gordon KC, Meyer B, Stevens N. A five-step "microskills" model of clinical teaching. *J Am Board Fam Pract* 1992; 5: 419–424.
15. Irby DM. What clinical teachers in medicine need to know. *Acad Med* 1994; 69(5): 333–342.
16. Carley S, Morris H, Kilroy D. Clinical teaching in emergency medicine: The board round at Hope Hospital emergency department. *Emerg Med J* 2007; 24: 659–661.

## CHAPTER 14

# Effective presentation skills

*Joseph R. Lex Jr.*
*Emergency Medicine, Temple University School of Medicine, Philadelphia,*
*PA, USA*

## Introduction

As a teacher of emergency medicine, you will sooner or later be asked to give a talk. Your reaction to that request will depend on a number of factors, including the didactic sessions you have heard throughout your education. You have been exposed to hundreds – if not thousands – of hours of talks during your career. Which ones are still clear in your memory? What made them exceptional? When you think about what makes a certain talk unforgettable, the features that almost certainly stand out are a knowledgeable teacher who was excited about the material and who was clearly eager for you to learn. That educator knew the material and projected enthusiasm about it. The talk was simple and well organized, which made it easy for you to take notes. There were only a few take-home points, and they were reiterated throughout and at the end of the talk. And the speaker finished at least 2 minutes early.

Why have you forgotten the hundreds of other talks you have attended? I will bet if you think about it you will recall poorly prepared speakers monotonously reading from slides with minuscule print and giving encyclopedic knowledge with no clear beginning, goal, or endpoint. That is what you must avoid if you want to be one of those memorable teachers your students speak about with admiration years after you have influenced them. This chapter will give you 10 principles you must follow to achieve that goal.

*Warning*: This chapter will *not* cover the use of PowerPoint® and other presentation materials. For that you will have to look elsewhere [1].

*Practical Teaching in Emergency Medicine*, 1st edition. Edited by R Rogers, A Mattu, M Winters & J Martinez. ©2009 Blackwell Publishing, ISBN: 9781405176224

## Rule #1: Know the type of talk you are giving

You will give two different types of talks through your career. The final goal for each type is the same: impart knowledge, change practice, and improve patient care and outcomes. The structure of each of these talks is very different.

### The core content talk

The first type is the so-called core content talk, which involves an apparently simple transfer of knowledge from a textbook chapter to a slideset to the mind of your learner. Initially, this looks easy – just copy-and-paste from the on-line version of the textbook and make up a bunch of slides. If you do this, it will be almost immediately apparent to your listeners that you have cobbled together endless facts which they can not possible absorb. They would be better off if you just photocopied the chapter and gave it to them to read during quiet time.

By definition, the core content talk must cover masses of material, much of which must be recognized or memorized. You can help your audience get a handle on the important material by dividing the essentials into bite-sized chunks.

For example, you are assigned the topic "Oral and Dental Emergencies." Outline your talk on paper before you ever go near the computer. Decide on the text you are going to use and see how the material is organized. Then divide the topic by anatomy, superficial to deep: lips, teeth, gums, tongue, palate, uvula, tonsils/peritonsillar area, and posterior oropharynx. Then talk about the important conditions affecting each of these structures and how to treat them: for example, lips: angular cheilitis (perlèche), herpes simplex (cold sores), lacerations and regional blocks, vermilion border, and so on. Next, talk about the teeth – teething, caries, 3rd molar pain, periapical abscess, pericoronitis, post-extraction pain and dry socket, post-extraction bleeding, chipped, loose, avulsed, and missing teeth. When you have finished your outline, then and only then should you start making slides, looking for illustrations, and so on.

If you follow this technique your talk will be organized so that your audience can take notes in outline format. Their notes at the end of the talk should look a lot like the outline you used to develop the talk. Your outline also makes for a natural handout – give it to your audience and let them fill in the blanks.

This type of talk supplements the written material, and your audience will benefit more by reading the assignment either before or after the presentation.

## The other talks

There are many other reasons to give a presentation. You may want to present the results of your own research, pass on a new message, clarify frequently confused information, motivate a change in practice, communicate a vision, or share a new and striking concept. The important thing to remember is that you must deliver information that the audience cannot get simply by reading a journal paper. And you always want to point your audience to additional learning resources.

In a 60-minute talk attended by 40 people, the cost is 40 human hours times the hourly value of each person's time plus the time spent traveling to hear the talk. If what you present could have been accomplished reading an article for 10 minutes while at the breakfast table or on the subway, you have wasted a *huge* amount of peoples' time.

The mark of a bad presenter is not necessarily withholding information, but giving too much without presorting and editing. This is not the time to become a human encyclopedia, inflicting fact after fact on a numbed group. Rather than say more, you should say less. Concentrate on delivering three to five major points. Your audience welcomes distilled information and a road map for learning. Again, think of the best presenters you have heard – they anticipated the question you might ask and answered it without prompting. That is the mark of a great teacher.

Another advantage of putting across a limited number of major points is that it makes your job of developing the talk easier. Instead of a 45-minute talk, you are now developing 3 or 4 or 5 talks, interrelated, but each only 9 to 15 minutes long. It is a lot easier to write a 10-minute talk than to develop a coherent 45-minute talk.

Now that you have a 10-minute block, write down the point you want to make in that segment. Only after you have the conclusion should you start developing that section. Your goal is to spend 9 minutes developing the argument made in the last 1 minute, much like a lawyer.

## Rule #2: Know your audience

If you speak only to residents, you know your audience. But what if you are invited to speak at another hospital, residency program, or unfamiliar setting? Do not assume you can give the same talk you give in front of a sympathetic crowd of people you work with daily. Find out who will be present – physicians, nurses, administrators, lay people. Are they all emergency physicians, or can you expect some trauma surgeons, family physicians, or hospitalists in the audience? What is the anticipated audience size? Why are they attending – required Continuing Medical Education? Do people primarily come for the free lunch? Is it a mandatory talk to meet some hospital or state requirement? Are there specific points that your host wants you to make? Can you expect disagreement from certain audience members? The more you know about your audience, the easier your job will be.

Also make sure that your cutting-edge technology is compatible with what is available at your speaking venue. Know whether you will be restricted to using a laptop at a podium or can freely wander and use a remote control.

## Rule #3: Know your ending

Why is this topic next? The end of the talk is the earliest part of the talk you should develop. Many talks are mediocre because they sputter to a halt with no warning, leaving the audience with a dissatisfied puzzled look. One of the most anticlimactic statements you can utter is "Well, I guess that's all I have." The end of the talk is your opportunity to sum-up and emphasize the points you want people to take home. Recap the three to five main points you will make, and tell people how to use them.

Another technique is to leave your audience with something extra to think about. You could finish by saying, "We've covered a lot of material today, but believe it or not there's more. Consider this ..." Take time to script and rehearse a strong, emotional concluding statement that leaves your audience with a vivid mental image.

Always end by saying "Thank you." If you do not cue your audience to the end, they may be confused (or annoyed). The social ritual of thanks, followed by applause, gives finality to your talk and comforts everyone. A question period may follow, but supply proper closure before starting the questions (see Rule #9: Set the ground rules).

## Rule #4: Know your beginning

After you have developed your ending, go back to the beginning. Giving a talk is like flying an airplane – the most difficult times are the take-off and the landing. The rest of the time, you should be on autopilot.

Start by introducing yourself, even if you have just been introduced. People are getting settled in and may have missed what someone said about you. Do not hesitate to tell people who you are, where you are from, and why you are giving this talk. It takes less than a minute and lets your audience see your confidence right from the beginning.

Memorize your opening, but not the whole talk. If you learn by rote the spiel for the first few slides, you will get a smooth start no matter how anxious or tired you are. It gives your nerves a chance to settle before you go into the autopilot portion of your talk. (If you do not feel that you can comfortably get to this state, see Rule #10: Getting over stage fright).

Tell the audience up front why they need to pay attention and why your talk is important to them. Examples: "I will give you the information you need to help prevent contrast-induced nephropathy in your patient" or "I will tell you about an injury which is the number one cause of successful litigation against emergency physicians." If you have not grabbed your listener's attention in the first few minutes, you may never do so later.

It is perfectly okay – and even encouraged – to give the conclusion at the beginning. Your audience hears it once at the beginning, a second time when you are in the middle of your talk, and a third time as you finish. You should even think about saying it a fourth time.

## Rule #5: Know your material

You have heard the statement before, and I will verify it for you: the best way to learn a subject is to teach it. Whether you tutor a group of Emergency Medical Technicians at a local fire station or you give a keynote presentation at an international gathering of hundreds or thousands, that principle stays the same. No matter how good your presentation skills may be, you will come up short if you do not know your topic backwards and forwards ... and sideways.

Anyone can read a bunch of slides. As an educator to be remembered, you must know your material well enough so that you can change things "on the fly," depending on the reactions from your audience. You can ad lib and improvise to meet the needs of your viewers as you see their responses: blank stares cause you to rephrase a statement, puzzled looks encourage you to find out where more explanation is needed. You are part editor, part director, and part actor. Rather than "lecture" you are involved in a running conversation with your listeners.

While preparing your talk, you will predictably learn something new about your subject. When you pass on that information to your audience, your enthusiasm will be apparent.

## Rule #6: Pay attention to your voice and tone

Quiet and dull never sold anything; your audience will not learn a thing if they are asleep. Talk just a little louder than you think is necessary. At first you will sound loud to yourself, but the audience interprets this as enthusiasm and authority. Your volume and projection must match your physical appearance or you will not look and or sound correct.

When starting, do not ask, "Can everybody hear me?" Rather, "Do I need to speak louder?" If somebody cannot hear you, they cannot answer your question.

While a bad speaker talks at the same speed, volume, and intensity throughout, a good speaker has a cadence and a volume that varies with the subject matter (odds ratio for falling asleep during talk with monotone presenter, 6.8) [2]. A good speaker emphasizes important words and ideas by speaking even louder, or by using a slow and deliberate voice, or by repeating a key concept. While we have been conditioned to think that silence ("dead air") is bad, a few seconds of quiet before and after a key point can drive it home effectively.

Organized communication comes from an organized mind. Give yourself permission to take as long as you need to develop what you will say next. You know the material, so trust yourself: stop thinking after you start a sentence. A poor speaker frequently rethinks a sentence once it is started, and what comes out is confused and uneven. When you do not know what to say next, be quiet: the audience is not going anywhere. You have a right to remain silent. You can even repeat the last thing you said in an effort to jog your memory; your audience will hear it as emphasis on whatever point you have just made.

It is not vanity to listen to yourself speak: it is essential. You will be your own most astute critic, picking up annoying tics and quirks you would never discover otherwise. Record and listen to yourself every chance you get. Count the number of times you start a sentence with "So..." or "By the way..." or "Basically...." Then count the number of times you end a sentence with "Okay?" as a question. You may be chagrined by your findings.

Practice pronouncing final syllables, and make sure that you form final consonants distinctly. Overdo it, since a large percentage of the population may have a hearing defect: think of them when you practice.

Many years ago when I was a radio announcer I was aghast when I first listened to my air-checks. I heard a "small market inflection," a slight upward inflection of the words at the end of a sentence in an effort to avoid monotone. You still hear it on most local community and college stations. As a polished speaker, you will avoid this vocal quirk.

Another thing I learned from radio is the "audience of one" technique. When you are sitting in a studio by yourself and speaking into a microphone, you try to speak to one person. You can translate this second-person singular technique to a roomful of people, but it takes practice. Rather than, "How many people use bedside ultrasound during the secondary trauma survey exams?" try saying "Do you do use bedside ultrasound during the secondary trauma survey exams?" It is a far more personable way to connect with your listeners as each person in the room hears the question as an individual, rather than as a crowd. Each time you ask a rhetorical question, look at one individual and phrase it to him or her. It takes some practice, but is a very powerful tool.

## Rule #7: Know your body language

A much-discussed study shows that students can accurately predict a teacher's ability to communicate effectively after watching a 30-second video clip of that teacher – with the sound turned off [3]. Even good teachers are not cognizant of how their body language and vocal nuances affect an audience's reception.

Fixing nonverbal behavior is not easy, and it is almost impossible to fix as you speak. You must concentrate on it during rehearsal. Slow down all your motions; concentrate on moving only one part of your body at a time very deliberately. Speaking is performance, and as a performance artist you should be aware of where your body is every minute. There is an athleticism and grace transmitted by the best speakers. It comes with practice.

Just as we get most of the information we retain from our visual sense, our strongest impressions of a speaker are often visual impressions. A gesture, whether intended or not, is apt to have as great an effect on listeners as the words you are speaking. Either make relevant, productive gestures or make none at all. Use your hands to make natural gestures, just as in normal conversation, but make them broader. Small gestures look tentative and uncertain when you are in front of a group. When you are not using your hands, keep them by your side. The fig leaf position with hands clasped in front of you looks defensive and gives the impression that you are apprehensive and lack certainty. It is okay to put your hands in your pockets occasionally, but do not keep them there for long as this impairs your ability to gesture naturally. And you will be tempted to play with keys, coins, or other items your hands may find.

Stand with your feet slightly apart – no more than the width of your shoulders. If your feet are too far apart, you will look confrontational. If your feet are too close together, you will look stiff and nervous, like you are standing at attention.

Facial expression is startlingly important. It has been reported that 7% of meaning is in the words that are spoken, 38% of meaning is in the way the words are said, and 55% of meaning is in facial expression, although this rule has been disputed. Enthusiasm is contagious. Let your audience know that you are committed to your ideas and excited about them; they will not only *hear* your enthusiasm, but they will *see* it in your body language and they will then feel it as well.

## Rule #8: Know your environment

If you speak in a room with a podium, ignore it except to avoid bumping into it or tripping over it. Move around the room. Make eye contact with everyone in the room at least twice during your talk. If the group is small, do it even more frequently. If there's a sturdy table, sit on it briefly. Your audience will be more comfortable with you if you seem comfortable with them. Movement gives the audience the impression that you are talking with them rather than at them.

If you are provided with a laser pointer, be very, very careful. I recommend not using it at all. Invest in an old-fashioned telescoping pointer. Think about the ways you have seen laser pointers used. Speakers have a tendency to "circle" items on their slides rather than point – and you have absolutely no idea what they want you to see. Do you still run your finger under the text when you read? If not, do not make your audience do the same. Put the laser down and no one will get hurt. If there is something you want to highlight, hold the laser light steady. But remember, every time you face the screen to use a laser pointer, you turn your back on your audience. Lastly, a "shaky" laser pointer may make the audience think you are nervous.

## Rule #9: Set the ground rules

Tell your audience how you will spend their time, and define how you will accept questions. Then leave time at the end to answer those questions.

Sometimes the hardest part is getting the first question, especially in a large audience where no one wants to be first. Break the ice by asking an easy "conversational" question related to your subject. Once the first audience member speaks, others will follow.

With an audience of 30 or more people, you should repeat the question so everyone knows exactly what question you are answering. This also gives you valuable time to think. You do not have to repeat the question verbatim; but make sure you restate the essential elements.

Avoid saying, "What a great question!" It often means, "I have an answer prepared for that," or implies that other questions maybe were not so great.

Look directly at the person who is asking you the question and make sure they are finished before you start your answer. Talk to the entire audience during your answer. If you direct your attention only to the questioner, you will lose the interest of the rest of your audience.

Finally, tell the audience when you are wrapping up: announce that you have time for only one more question. Be specific.

Another tactic is to finish the body of the lecture, announce that you will take a few questions, and then summarize the main points of your talk. That method allows you to conclude with a powerful finish and walk away to applause. Do not let the question session be anticlimactic, occurring while most of your audience is getting up to leave.

## Rule #10: Deal with the stage fright [4]

> When you suffer an attack of nerves you are being attacked by the nervous system. What chance has a man got against a system?
>
> Russell Hoban

Although stage fright can mean many things to many people, the most common symptoms are dry mouth, tight throat, sweaty, cold or shaky hands, nausea, tachycardia, shaky knees, and trembling lips. As per the Diagnostic and Statistical Manual of Mental Disorders (DSM-IV), many of these are identical to features found in anxiety and panic attacks.

Think of fear as your friend. When you are nervous about speaking, you will be more conscious of your posture and breathing. Excess adrenaline heightens your energy, dilates your pupils, and improves your reflexes. These side effects actually make you look healthier and more physically attractive.

The trickiest time is before your start. If you know your material, the stage fright goes away once you start speaking. How many times have you complimented someone on a job well done and found out afterwards that they were extremely nervous? Remember that nervousness does not show one-tenth as much as it feels.

Not everyone reacts the same to stage fright; there is also no universal guaranteed fix for stage fright. Many techniques are recommended by many public speakers; you may need to experiment to find the ones right for you. First and foremost, stay in shape; public speaking is an athletic endeavor. Arrive at the site you will speak early enough to find out where everything is located in the room. Engage in conversation with attendees, and intently listen to what they are saying. If you speak from notes, hide cartoons or pictures of your children (or grandchildren) in the papers. Use eye contact so you feel less isolated. Find the friendliest faces in the audience and talk to them until you relax. You can even joke about your nervousness.

## Now that you have got it all together: Practice, practice, practice

Amateurs practice until they get it right; professionals practice until they cannot get it wrong. There are very few people who are "naturals" when it comes to public speaking. Speaking is just like tennis or golf; it is a physical activity that requires hard work and a lot of practice. Just like your golf or tennis game, your speaking style will suffer with inactivity: use it or lose it. Speaking opportunities are abundant, so start speaking every chance you get. Volunteer to speak at local hospitals, fire stations, service organizations, nursing schools – the opportunities are boundless.

Rehearsal is much more that just going through the presentation time after time; it is preparation time that simulates the actual speaking conditions as closely as possible. Plan how you will verbally emphasize key phrases and ideas, especially points that you are going to repeat. Do not try to rehearse specific gestures, as they invariably come across as phony.

Rehearsal means speaking out loud. Internal language is different from spoken language, and merely reciting the material to yourself is not an effective method of rehearsal. Author Herman Hesse said, "Everything becomes a little different as soon as it is spoken out loud." Suddenly the redundancies, the uneven flow, the unclear conclusions reveal themselves. Internal language is silent, grammatically condensed, and semantically condensed [5].

Feedback from an audience knowledgeable about your topic is also helpful, but not always available. Getting feedback is tricky, and you may want to prepare your test audience by asking them to give both good and bad things about your talk. Feedback should be specific and focus on things that you can change. To receive feedback, you must be receptive to it. No one likes criticism, because it always hurts at least a little bit. But think about how – or whether – to incorporate this feedback into improving your style or presentation.

Nothing can take the place of recording and listening to your practice sessions. Get a tape recorder, mp3 recorder, or figure out how to use the recording function on your computer or PDA. First go through your talk without an audience, speak in a normal conversational voice into the recording device, then listen: you will learn a lot from this first playback. Then do a second run-through; this time concentrate on staying close to your time limit and on making smooth transitions from one point to the next. On your third recording, have at least one other person in the room, stand up, and speak loudly and clearly just as you will in the actual situation.

Complete your final practice session before the day of your presentation. You will get virtually no benefit from last-minute practice. Instead, use the few hours just before you speak to reflect on the concepts and major theme of your presentation.

## Summary points: Top 10 tips for successful speaking

- Know the type of talk you are giving
- Know your audience
- Begin with end in mind – know your ending well
- Know your beginning
- Know your material very well
- Pay attention to your voice and tone
- Know and pay attention to your body language
- Get familiar with your speaking environment
- Set the ground rules for your audience
- Consider stage fright and practice, practice, practice

## Conclusion

Being a good presenter is not a one-time event. Review a recording every few months to check your progress. Listen to good speakers every chance you get, whether in person or from commercial Continuing Medical Education programs. Then listen again and concentrate on what makes that speaker effective – the voice, enthusiasm, mannerisms, and ability to put across motivating ideas.

Your personal style of public speaking may not be the same as anybody you know, but there is no unique model for a successful speaker. The yardstick for a good presenter is simply effectiveness in getting your message across.

To speak like an expert, get up there and say something that will make your audience lose track of time and forget everything else in the world except what you are telling them. Every appearance must be your best, as it might be the last thing people remember about you.

## References

1. LaPorte RE, Linkov F, Villasenor T, *et al.* Papyrus to PowerPoint (P 2 P): metamorphosis of scientific communication. *BMJ* 2002; 325(7378): 1478–1481.
2. Rockwood K, Hogan DB, Patterson CJ. Incidence of and risk factors for nodding off at scientific sessions. *CMAJ* 2004; 171(12): 1443–1445.
3. Anbady N, Rosenthal R. Half a minute: Predicting teacher evaluation from thin slices of nonverbal behavior and physical attractiveness. *J Pers Soc Psychol* 1993; (64): 431.
4. www.public-speaking.org/public-speaking-stagefright-article.htm
5. Zak-Dance CC, Dance FEX: Speaking Your Mind: Private Thinking and Public Speaking. Kendall Hunt Pub Co, 1993.

# CHAPTER 15

# Small group discussion skills

*Matthew D. Deibel[1], Mary Jo Wagner[2]*
[1]*Emergency Care Center, Covenant HealthCare, Saginaw, MI; Program in Emergency Medicine, Michigan State University College of Human Medicine, East Lansing, MI, USA*
[2]*Synergy Medical Education Alliance/Michigan State University, Emergency Medicine Residency Program, Saginaw, MI; Program in Emergency Medicine, Michigan State University College of Human Medicine, East Lansing, MI, USA*

## Small group discussions

Discussions in a small group setting are remarkably effective educational techniques commonly used in medical educational curriculum. Successful in many different settings, small group discussions are likely to occur on change of shift rounds, while teaching ACLS or doing simulation training. Any large group can be divided up to accomplish the goals and gain the advantage of a small group discussion. The key to a valuable small group discussion is just that – making it a discussion. The effective leader will act more like a facilitator in encouraging the learners to come up with their own answers, thus developing a deeper understanding of the material. Trainees learn how to work together efficiently in small groups, an essential skill for any physician.

## Benefits of small group discussions

Small group discussions allow the trainee to utilize a higher level of learning [1]. There is a continuum of learning that begins with basic knowledge and comprehension, and then progresses through application, analysis, synthesis, and evaluation [2]. These latter

*Practical Teaching in Emergency Medicine*, 1st edition. Edited by R Rogers, A Mattu, M Winters & J Martinez. ©2009 Blackwell Publishing, ISBN: 9781405176224

processes are essential in the training of a physician and this is where the discussion format excels.

Small group discussions give the student the opportunity to be more involved in learning, thus increasing retention. Studies show that an active learner is a more effective learner and the chances of retention are much higher [3, 4]. The trade-off for this educational style is that less material can be covered in the same amount of time compared to lecture. However, as the learner is forced to discuss and conceptualize the topic, a deeper and more permanent understanding develops. Research shows that group interaction helps stimulate student learning by integrating new information onto existing knowledge [5]. This framework develops a more global understanding and improves long-term retention [2].

One of the biggest gains during this dynamic process is from interactions with others. Here trainees learn to think critically on their feet while discussing ideas and absorbing input from multiple sources to come up with a plan. In addition to the increased medical knowledge, interpersonal and communication skills are improved as the group works together. These same skills are invaluable to the learners as they progress through their training, specifically in the emergency department.

## When to use small groups

Small groups in emergency medicine are beneficial for almost any educational objective, but this technique is most effective for higher levels of learning like application, analysis, synthesis, and evaluation. Basic knowledge and comprehension are best taught in a lecture format or as assigned reading before a discussion. To be effective, a large contingent of faculty members must be available to assist with each small group session. In addition, there must be enough space and time for a small group session to proceed naturally.

### Developing a skill set

A small group discussion is an excellent way to reinforce information that was provided in an initial overview given by lecture or assigned reading. One example of this would be with a skill such as reading electrocardiograms (ECGs). When the basic knowledge has already been provided, the interaction time with the instructor can be spent in discussion and answering questions rather than passing on rote facts.

## Teaching procedures

A small group is usually the best way to teach a procedure. An important aspect of demonstrating a procedure is to allow each learner to see the appropriate anatomical landmarks and each piece of equipment while its use is explained. For instance, in learning how to place a central line, a small group of trainees can observe and discuss each step around a model more effectively than during a lecture with slides. Having a senior house officer as the group leader who is teaching the procedure and leading the discussion will also reinforce the procedural skills for this trainee.

## Case-based learning

Individual cases can be utilized to practice this teaching concept. A case or cases, with associated questions can be given in advance of the discussion. All the learners develop their own answers before meeting, allowing time for those having less background knowledge of the topic to preview the subject matter. Then the case is discussed in the small group. This is particularly appropriate for students or junior house officers.

## Literature review

Breakout sessions may be used at a journal club or literature review session, with small group discussions facilitating the different levels of understanding of each group. As a large group, the entire training program may discuss the same articles with different trainees presenting an article and then all participants discussing global strengths and weakness. Then the house officers can be broken down into smaller groups based on level, to concentrate more on learning specific skills (e.g. reviewing the basic statistics.) The involvement of every member of the group creates a more meaningful and active learning environment for the trainee.

## Role-playing

Role-playing is an effective technique done with small group discussions used in training emergency medicine specialists. Generally, a case is presented and the group of learners then approaches the case with another member of the group acting as the patient. This is most effective when the story has been developed in advance and the person acting as the patient understands his role prior to starting. Time should be given afterward for the learners to analyze themselves, each other, and then dissect how the case progressed.

As with most feedback sessions, the group should be encouraged to focus on each other's strengths before pointing out deficiencies. This role-playing and subsequent small group discussion affords trainees opportunities to work through critical and stressful situations in their minds before being overwhelmed in the emergency department.

In particular, role-playing is useful in evaluating the trainee's ability to effectively communicate in difficult cases. Frequently used role-playing sessions might include giving bad news, dealing with an angry parent, or helping calm an agitated psychiatric patient. With a structured case, similar communication issues challenge each student and a faculty member in the small group can formally assess their performance. This can be a powerful tool for determining competency in the areas that normally have less objective evaluation techniques (e.g. communication skills).

### Problem-based learning

Problem-based learning (PBL) has recently been gaining more attention as it is being used more frequently in U.S. medical school education. It is different from simple small group discussions in that participants are encouraged to use self-directed learning skills [6]. The student is responsible for deciding what needs to be learned, and then learning it [1]. This is done in a group setting where an open-ended clinical scenario is proposed. The students then need to analyze it, formulating, and prioritizing key learning objectives from the case. They then disband to collect the needed information and regroup after some days to discuss the findings [6]. This interaction gives the learners a sense of ownership of the new knowledge. Benefit has been shown in undergraduate education and in the first two years of medical school. It has not been looked at closely in postgraduate medical training programs. This chapter does not focus on PBL, but the interested reader can review other sources that talk about PBL in medicine (Table 15.1) [1, 5, 6].

## Characteristics and techniques of a good facilitator

### Facilitator characteristics

A skilled facilitator is necessary to achieve the discussion objectives and maintain cohesion of the small group during the task [1] (See Table 15.1). Discussions, by nature, are unpredictable and good facilitator must be spontaneous and creative [2]. Being comfortable

**Table 15.1** How to be a good facilitator.

| Characteristics to develop |
| --- |
| Spontaneity and creativity |
| Comfort with ambiguity |
| Good sense of humor |
| Enthusiasm for learning |
| Approachability |
| Solid clinical knowledge |
| Acknowledge limitations |

| Techniques to master |
| --- |
| Preparation |
| Restraint |
| Questioning |
| Summarizing |
| Brainstorming |
| Adjusting tension level |

with ambiguity and differing opinions helps, along with a good sense of humor.

Enthusiasm for learning and respect for the learner are also necessary traits for a facilitator. Learners clearly respond better to faculty who are approachable and appear interested. Trainees look to someone who is knowledgeable, a good clinician that is confident in his or her clinical skills. At the same time, in two different studies of effective teachers, students clearly appreciated faculty who would acknowledge when they did not know the answer either [7, 8]. This facilitates the discussion as the group looks up the information together.

## Techniques

### Preparation

Some successful lecturers do poorly as discussion facilitators because they do not understand the unique preparation and techniques required in this learning environment [2]. The faculty leader must first believe that the small group discussion is a valid and powerful teaching method. Preparation time is similar to organizing a lecture. Along with gathering necessary material, the learners' knowledge base must be assessed and specific goals for the session need to be clearly defined. It is important for the facilitator to remember that not as much detail can be covered in a group discussion as in lecture. Without planning for a discussion, an urgency to cover all the material develops and instead of allowing the free exchange of ideas and deeper learning, many teachers then revert to the classic lecture format [9].

## Restraint

The facilitator will likely have the answer that the group is looking for, but specifically providing this knowledge defeats the purpose of the group discussion. In fact, an effective facilitator need not be a content expert, as an energetic leader with an understanding of the group interactions is more valuable than a less dynamic leader with medical proficiency expertise in the subject [6]. Having expertise in the particular topic may even be disadvantageous to the group as one might have a tendency to return to the lecture mode. Still, the faculty member may want to submit an occasional, thoughtful personal experience for everyone's learning and to generate further discussion.

## Questioning

There are three reasons a facilitator uses questions: to initiate discussion, to encourage participation, and to keep the discussion on track [2]. Questions can be open or closed, but always need to be specific. Open questions will broaden a topic, while closed questions are used to drill down on a specific idea. Enthusiasm for all answers, not just the correct ones, will increase participation. The leader must be comfortable with silence and not pass a question on to another student until there has been plenty of time to ponder the answer. Questions from group members directed to the leader should be put back out to the group.

## Summarizing

Summarization is frequently used to emphasize every major topic and to regain the group's focus as needed. This is a brief statement that includes comments made by multiple group members. By creating a rhythm of questions and answers, with frequent summarization, the facilitator can help lead the group to achieve "moments of greater understanding" [2].

## Brainstorming

The key to brainstorming is to hold judgment until after all ideas are generated. Encourage the learners to improve on their ideas by combining and building on them. Time is given afterward for evaluation. In emergency medicine, this is commonly used in developing a differential diagnosis in a case-based learning scenario.

### Adjusting tension level

All verbal interactions are associated with a certain tone, level of tension, or ambiance [2]. The moderator's goal is to keep the group at a moderate tone. If the atmosphere is too stressful, then group members will feel inhibited and not easily contribute. If the mood is too lenient, then the discussion can become too casual and unproductive. The tenor in professional settings is usually too high, so the moderator should approach the discussion with a comfortable, conversational tone [2]. Preparation is paramount to actively adjust the tone of a group (Table 15.2).

## Getting started with a small group discussion

### Establishing goals

Before embarking on organized small group discussions, goals for the educational exercises should be defined. This will likely include learning objectives with the specific key points of knowledge, for example, the treatment protocols for acute asthma. The group members must also know that active participation of all members is required.

### Sizing the group for discussion

Some forethought should be given to how the group should be organized to accomplish the established goals. Groups of 5–8 people seem to be ideal for most small group discussions in emergency medicine. A larger group can be broken into smaller segments for discussion. If a larger group is kept together, a clear facilitation plan is needed so everyone has an equal opportunity to contribute.

### Choosing a seating arrangement

While this may not seem important, the seating arrangement is directly related to how the individual will participate. Each member of the group must be in a position to see everyone else. A rectangular table would not allow this as well as a circular one, or even just a cluster of chairs. The group can assemble in pairs around a circle for one-on-one discussion or role-play. A larger group may have an inner circle that discusses a topic, while an outer circle listens in [9].

The position of the facilitator is particularly important. If the facilitator is positioned at the head of the table or is at a focus point in the group, it is more likely that the group will fall back into a lecturing format. This can be minimized by having the facilitator either sitting in the group as one of the members or by wandering away from the group at times, returning long enough to ensure the group is still on task. Trainees may still look to the facilitator for answers each time instead of looking to each other. The facilitator should avoid the temptation to answer and instead make eye contact with one of the students, rephrasing the question if needed.

## Selecting materials

The instructor must determine which materials should be given prior to the session for the students to review. Again, small group discussions are not a good place to introduce new knowledge. Therefore a chapter in the assigned textbook, a series of journal articles or case summaries may need to be assigned before the discussion. Literature review articles should be chosen based on academic interest and ability to generate discussion. Alternatively, a formal lecture could precede the discussion. The appropriate material and format depends on the type of small group session planned.

Then there are times when the materials are more appropriately held until the start of the discussion. Oral examination cases are a good example of this. After one learner works through a case, the group then discusses the specific clinical situation. Case-based scenarios are usually given in advance but may be held until the discussion. These can also be taken from actual interesting cases, available educational material, or simply put together by a faculty member. Procedural cases may simply describe the procedure or teach using hands-on simulation. In all cases, the level of difficulty must be challenging enough to keep everyone's interest, while being simple enough to cover in one sitting.

## Setting the rules and expectations

It is important that everyone is aware of what is expected of him or her. Each house officer needs to come prepared if background material is given prior to the small group session. Each person is expected to contribute to the discussion. The initial session must also emphasize that people need to be given the opportunity to express their opinions without interruption and that critical comments should be kept to a minimum. Encouragement and praise for something said or done well should precede constructive criticism. Everyone needs to be aware of the evaluation process from the beginning. Time allowed must be clearly defined with a set start and end time.

**Table 15.2** Techniques for success – 10 things to get started.

---

**1. Determine the type of small group**
Opportunities exist in teaching procedures and skill sets, discussing cases, practicing oral boards, reviewing articles at breakout sessions, role-playing scenarios, and working through simulations.

**2. Establish goals**
Define specific points of learning, including the importance of teamwork.

**3. Size the group**
Decide the number of participants based on the type of small group. Break up a large group into smaller segments as appropriate.

**4. Arrange seating**
Allow everyone to see each other, with the facilitator not sitting in a lead position.

**5. Select materials**
Depending on the type of small group, readings may be given for individual review before the discussion. Material used in the discussion must be challenging enough to generate a conversation, yet simple enough to cover in the allotted time.

**6. Set the expectations**
Everyone must contribute, with the evaluation process transparent. Encouragement and praise should always dominate any constructive criticism.

**7. Facilitate the discussion**
Avoid lecturing and stay enthusiastic and approachable. Pause before contributing to allow students to speak first.

**8. Ensure equal contributions**
Check individual preparation where appropriate. Call on specific people by name to add a comment as needed.

**9. Stay on task**
Prepare ahead of time. Knowing what is to be covered will help redirect the discussion if the group is moving off course. Realize not as much material will be covered as in a lecture format, but the retention is higher.

**10. Assess the discussion**
Trainees may be evaluated on preparation, participation, and performance. The group leader should receive feedback to enhance facilitation skills.

---

## Challenges and solutions of small group discussions

### Keeping the small group in a discussion

There is a tendency in small group discussions for the facilitator to talk too much and convert the experience into a lecture format. This can be minimized by principles discussed earlier. In particular, adequate preparation, proper seating, and specific questions with a tolerance for silence will help keep the group in a discussion.

### Getting all to participate

If there is material that needs to be reviewed prior to the discussion, then the members of the group should hold individuals accountable for their preparation. The faculty member can accomplish this by having all participants show their notes or he may give a small quiz. Some members may seem shy and not participate as much, so a skillful facilitator must call individuals by name at times for their opinion to help engage them in the group discussion. Strong positive reinforcement is most important with those that contribute the least.

### Preventing one participant from dominating the discussion

While this person may or may not have good intentions, he or she must be reminded that this is a discussion. Starting with subtle reminders by asking others to voice their opinions, the facilitator can refer back to this person only after other members of the group have spoken. If there is still a problem, then the group leader may thank the individual for all his or her input, but then gently ask that he or she give others a chance to contribute first. Alternately, the moderator can cut across the individual's talk with a summarizing statement and then direct a question to another student.

### Staying on task

This is where the facilitator is most useful in keeping the topic clear and the discussion focused. Some side discussion may be beneficial, especially as the group delves deeper into one aspect of the topic that interests them. If the facilitator sees that the group is moving off course completely, then it is up to him or her to get the group back on discussion. Summarizing what has been covered so far and bringing up the next question for the group to discuss will usually get the discussion back on course. Adequate preparation, from both the trainees and the facilitator, will also help keep everyone on task.

## Assessing the discussion

An important aspect to a successful small group discussion is assessment. In evaluating the student, a faculty member should focus on knowledge transfer, not solely on the correct answer. This may only be an oral assessment, but it is important that they receive this feedback. Hearing this immediate feedback will help solidify key concepts and reinforce the individual strengths and weaknesses as a participant in a group.

Individually, students can be evaluated on preparation, participation, and performance. Preparation can be assessed by something as simple as an opinion from the faculty member or as formal as a quiz prior to the discussion to ensure that the required reading was completed. If questions were assigned prior to a discussion, everyone can be asked to show their answers, if only to see if they were completed.

Assessing participation can be accomplished by keeping track of who contributes to the discussion. If lack of participation is a general problem, then individual involvement should be documented. Having every trainee rate each other's level of participation at the end of a discussion is another powerful assessment tool. This peer feedback is an excellent summary to include in a house officer's educational portfolio or file.

Performance is the final part of the student's assessment. This looks more at individual answers given by the learner. Performance may also include the student's use of insightful questions and ability to bring up additional points of discussion.

Feedback for facilitator performance can be instantaneous at the session, or part of the overall faculty evaluation. Either way, it is important for the faculty member to also get feedback on what he does well as a facilitator and what he needs to work on. Feedback should include his ability to keep the discussion flowing smoothly along with the characteristics and techniques reviewed earlier.

## Conclusion

The small group discussion is an effective educational teaching tool in many environments. Increased participation in the learning process can increase interest and retention in a subject area. Useful for in depth discussions of previously taught concepts, the small group can provide a setting for reflective questioning and critical thinking. One of the most important aspects of a successful small group is the preparation and skill of the facilitator, who moves the discussion along while allowing all members equal participation. With the proper groundwork, enthusiastic learner participation, and helpful feedback at the end of the session, the small group discussions will be the favorite learning mode of a program's learners and teachers.

---

### Summary points

- Small groups allow for in depth discussion of a topic
- A key to success is a prepared and skilled facilitator
- Enthusiastic participation by the learners increases the small group's effectiveness

---

# References

1. Crosby J. Learning in small groups and problem-based learning. In: Sweet J, Uttly S, Taylor I, eds. *Medial, Dental & Veterinary Education: Learning in Small Groups and Problem-based Learning*, Kogan Page, Sterling, VA, 2003: 101–121.
2. Whitman N, Schwenk T. *A Handbook for Group Discussion Leaders*. University of Utah School of Medicine, Salt Lake City, 1999.
3. Cooper JL, MacGregor J, Smith KA, Robinson P. Implementing small-group instruction: insights from successful practitioners. In: *New directions for teaching and learning*, Jossey-Bass Publishers (2000); 81: 63–76.
4. Johnson JP, Mighten A. A comparison of teaching strategies: lecture notes combined with structured group discussion versus lecture only. *J Nurs Educ* 2005; 44: 319–322.
5. Visschers-Pleijers AJ, Dolmans DH, Leng BA, Wolfhagen IH, Vleuten CP. Analysis of verbal interactions in tutorial groups: a process study. *Med Educ* 2006; 40: 129–137.
6. Kilroy DA. Problem based learning. *Emerg Med J* 2004; 21: 411–413.
7. Bandiera G, Lee S, Tiberius R. Creating effective learning in today's emergency departments: how accomplished teachers get it done. *Ann Emerg Med* 2005; 45: 253–261.
8. Steinert Y. Student perceptions of effective small group teaching. *Med Educ* 2004; 38: 286–293.
9. Jaques D. ABC of learning and teaching in medicine: teaching small groups. *BMJ* 2003; 326: 492–494.

# CHAPTER 16

# Faculty development as a guide for becoming a better teacher

*Gloria J. Kuhn*
*Department of Emergency Medicine, Wayne State University, Detroit, MI, USA*

## Defining faculty development

Faculty development programs may be defined as "Those programs which provide the intellectual tools and skills to assist faculty members in accomplishing their academic goals." The Professional and Organizational Network for Higher Education divides faculty development programs into those focusing on (1) improving teaching, (2) those developing the individual as a scholar and professional and include grant writing, and writing manuscripts for publication, and (3) those focusing on the faculty member as a person and would examine stress, well being, or interpersonal relations (www.podnetwork.org accessed 7/15/07) [1].

Most organized faculty development programs have elements that include not only teaching but information on scholarly activity and professional development as successful academic physicians will need all of this knowledge and skills. Indeed, the goal in many university faculty development programs is to educate physicians who intend to specialize in medical education within the medical school setting [2].

With that in mind, this chapter will discuss faculty development programs and resources to assist faculty in developing the skills and abilities needed for (1) effective and efficient clinical teaching,

*Practical Teaching in Emergency Medicine*, 1st edition. Edited by R Rogers, A Mattu, M Winters & J Martinez. ©2009 Blackwell Publishing, ISBN: 9781405176224

(2) methods for customizing an individualized comprehensive faculty development program to enhance clinical teaching, and (3) documentation of expertise and productivity in teaching for purposes of promotion.

## Practicing in an academic setting

Some academic environments, often, but not entirely in community settings, have two types of faculty: (1) those physicians wishing to restrict their time almost solely to the clinical practice of medicine coupled with bedside teaching and supervision, with delivery of an occasional formal teaching presentation and (2) those who wish to become core faculty with requirements that they teach, engage in scholarly activity, and provide service to their institution and specialty. Other academic environments, often in university settings, require that all faculty fulfill the obligations of teaching, scholarly activity (defined as research in many universities), and service. It is critical for young faculty to decide in which type of environment they wish to practice as this decision will drive the type of faculty development they need and the kinds of activities in which they engage.

Excellence in teaching is not enough for success or promotion in a university setting. Faculty must demonstrate scholarly activity. Although, on the surface, all universities and medical schools seem similar in their requirements, they vary widely in how they define and value various activities and the amount and types of activities which are acceptable to ensure promotion. This is important because the culture of the institution drives these value systems. A faculty member only wanting to practice clinical medicine and teach will not do well in an environment and culture which emphasizes and values research and acquisition of grants to support that research. Fortunately, the university culture is slowly changing so that the definition of scholarly activity is being broadened beyond "discovery of new knowledge" as medical school deans realize that they need clinicians to teach medical students and residents and provide clinically generated revenues to help support the medical schools [3, 4].

Community settings put much less emphasis on research and scholarly activity but even there core faculty must engage in scholarly activity to satisfy the needs of the program to create a scholarly learning environment for residents, deliver a well thought out curriculum, teach effectively, and to fulfill the requirements of residency review committees for scholarship from faculty. For further details see the Accreditation Council for Graduate Medical Education (ACGME) website http://www.acgme.org/acWebsite/RRC. It is for all of the above reasons that faculty development programs have a diversity of goals and teach many topics in addition to "how to teach."

## Clinicians as teachers

The expert clinical teacher needs a deep knowledge of the practice of emergency medicine, the desire to teach, and the will to learn how to teach. Most physicians have the first two prerequisites: the knowledge of emergency medicine and the desire to teach. Because every physician has been exposed to teachers for many years it is often assumed that by emulating their behaviors excellence in teaching is assured. But becoming an expert in teaching requires more than copying behavior, it requires an understanding of what makes teaching effective, how people learn, and developing your own style to become an effective teacher. Wilkerson and Irby have noted, " … whereas it was once assumed that a competent basic or clinical scientist would naturally be an effective teacher, it is now acknowledged that preparation for teaching is essential" [5].

## Setting goals

The first step in planning an academic career is to set goals as these will lay the foundation for academic activities. Both short- and long-term goals should be set. Short-term goals should help in attaining the long-term goals but long-term goals can and do change during a career. If the long-term goal is to practice medicine and teach, then programs or courses emphasizing teaching should be chosen. If the long-term goal is a broad academic career, faculty development programs with a variety of topics will be the best choice. Faculty in all academic settings need to become experts in bedside and didactic teaching.

The first prerequisite of teaching is content knowledge. Physicians, in general, are extremely knowledgeable and those who want to teach within their institution or on a national level need to know more than the audience. Many of those recognized for excellence in teaching have developed expertise in a particular subject that interested them so that they have depth of knowledge. Find topics to teach that you find fascinating, thus encouraging investment of time to gain expertise in the subject matter. Once enough content is obtained (true mastery can take a lifetime of on going study) it is time to develop expertise in one or more teaching methods.

Most think of teaching as either bedside teaching or giving a lecture. There are a number of award winning emergency physicians who are nationally recognized for their excellence in giving presentations. What distinguishes these lecturers is not only their depth of knowledge about the subject(s) they are teaching, but also their ability to catch and keep the attention of their audiences. That requires gaining skills in public speaking and use of a variety of instructional strategies to make lecturing interactive.

Lecturing is, however, the tip of the iceberg for educators. Emergency physicians are branching out into many venues. Constructing self-instruction modules for independent learning, which can include various types of multimedia, is an area ripe for further development in emergency medicine.

Distance education is a methodology of teaching that delivers instruction effectively to millions of people each year and is used all over the world. A number of emergency physicians have created websites containing either education materials or information pertaining to clinical medicine pertinent to emergency medicine. These sites include EMedHome.com and eMedicine which have multiple contributors and thousands of "hits" per day. There are websites to teach evidence-based medicine (EBM), radiology, and electrocardiography to name a few, some started by individual physicians and others the products of emergency physicians in interest groups (Table 16.1).

All of these modalities of teaching, some of which include multimedia, small-group discussions, distance education with construction of web sites, simulation training, and other educational methods and formats, will challenge educators to become proficient in skills and obtain knowledge beyond how to "make slides" or "teach in the department."

## Developing a customized program

Many medical educators, at least early in their careers, wish to construct a self-study program. This often consists of reading articles on teaching and attending lectures or short workshops of several days' length on teaching. Constructing a "curriculum" will allow a

**Table 16.1** Medical education Websites of emergency physicians.

| | | |
|---|---|---|
| EMedHome.com (Rick Nunez) | Medical information and CME available (requires a fee) | http://www.emedhome.com/ |
| eMedicine | Medical information | http://www.emedicine.com/ |
| National Center for Emergency Medicine Informatics | Information on EBM | http://www.ncemi.org/ |
| Radiology (Joshua Broder) | Images, quizzes, free registration | www.empacs.org |
| General Emergency Medicine (Scott Weingart) | Information on various topics on emergency medicine | http://www. emcrit.org/ |
| SAEM EBM Interest Group | Variety of information and topics related to EBM | http://www.ebem.org/index.php |

systematic approach to filling gaps in knowledge, gaining necessary skills, and avoiding redundancy. This does not have to be extremely involved, early on, but at the very least should include techniques for bedside teaching, formal presentations including lecturing, facilitated small-group discussion, procedural workshops, and mentoring. Other skills to be mastered include public speaking, making effective handouts and slides, and searching the literature, not only in the National Library of Medicine but within the literature on education and psychology (for this a librarian is an invaluable resource). A very "quick and dirty" way of doing this is to look at some of the formal faculty development programs that exist and pick and choose the areas of knowledge that pertain to bedside and didactic teaching as well as other areas of desired knowledge and skills.

After compiling the customized curriculum it is advisable to show it to a more experienced colleague or an educator to determine if it includes everything needed. It is important to remember that learning what is in the customized curriculum may take a number of years. Once the needed knowledge and skills are determined it is time to find resources.

**Table 16.2** Characteristics of successful speakers.

| Speaker | Content |
| --- | --- |
| Voice, tone, rapidity of speech | Organization and amount |
| Posture and movements | Explanations and answers provided to questions |
| Body language | Use of multimedia |
| Interaction with audience | |

One method of learning is to watch others when attending a presentation, especially by a well known and successful teacher. To use this method it is necessary to concentrate on the *teaching style* and *strategies* rather than on the content of the presentation. A number of questions should be asked about the speaker (Table 16.2). Use the same analysis to decide what is not done well. Finally, determine what you can use and what you will discard from the strategies and teaching style of the presentation. Decide what you can incorporate into your teaching as you develop your own style.

## Finding resources

### Professional societies

Joining professional societies can provide many benefits. Perhaps one of the most important is "networking". Getting to know others in academic emergency medicine will allow you to ask questions, learn what is important in building a career and, perhaps most important, it is a way to "become involved". Committee members are chosen from those who are known and who have come to meetings of a committee in the past. Being at a meeting and volunteering to work on a project with others helps you become known and allows you to begin to develop expertise in an area, making you an ideal candidate for a future project or committee assignment. After you are known you will find yourself invited to write book chapters, participate on panels and committees, or be part of a research project.

Emergency medicine educators will find it of value to join the Council of Residency Directors for Emergency Medicine (CORD). This society is open to educators in emergency medicine. The departmental chair or program director need only submit the educator's name and pay the small membership fee. This gives access to the CORD list serve where members are constantly discussing matters of education and which give faculty access to a "network" of information and philosophy on a large number of educational subjects. This is the "oral wisdom" of educators in emergency medicine who have a wealth of practical experience. Anyone can pose a question and there are always a broad number of topics discussed. Membership in CORD is not necessary to attend the Academic Assembly which is the annual faculty development program sponsored by CORD (discussed later).

The Society for Academic Emergency Medicine (SAEM) is also very popular with emergency medicine educators. The society publishes the journal, *Academic Emergency Medicine*, which carries articles on education as well as articles on clinical medicine. It has multiple committees and task forces, many of which are concerned with academic matters. It also sponsors a number of interest groups, many devoted to academic activities. Joining an interest group in an area in which you are interested, such as, EBM, simulation, or undergraduate education will allow you to meet others with interests similar to your own and can be very valuable.

Both the American College of Emergency Physicians (ACEP) and American Association of Emergency Medicine (AAEM) have committees, panels, and interest groups, some of which are involved in academic matters. Joining one of these organizations will have similar benefits such as networking and helping you become known.

## Printed materials

The most common and convenient method of learning is independent, using printed books, monographs, and journal articles on teaching. The problem is not to find resources but to find *good* resources that will supply (1) the information you need in (2) a format you want, and (3) within your budgeted time. A place to begin a literature search in journals is through Medline, sponsored by the National Library of Medicine and National Institutes of Health. A librarian can help you refine your search so you can find exactly what you need for either content or teaching methodologies and strategies.

There are a number of journals devoted to medical education including Academic Medicine, Medical Educator, Medical Researcher, and Teaching and Learning in Medicine. All have articles on medical education. The *British Medical Journal* is a very practical source of information. Specialty and subspecialty journals also have articles on teaching including, of course, those in emergency medicine. The *Canadian Medical Association Journal* and the *Journal of General Internal Medicine* frequently will have articles on teaching and faculty development.

Some of the authors who are known for writing on medical education include Geoffrey Norman, Glenn Reghr, Kevin Eva, Howard Barrows, and George Bordage. They write on a mixture of topics including how people learn, the psychology of clinical decision making and problem-based learning. These are just a very few authors but can get you started. Some useful articles and books on faculty development and teaching are listed in the Suggested Reading List at the end of this chapter.

## Online materials

The internet is a wealth of information, some good and useful, while other materials will not help. Mary Jo Wagner compiled a list of internet resources related to faculty development and medical education which she presented at the Advanced Teaching Fellowship sponsored by ACEP. Sam Luber listed all of those online resources at www.emergencymeducation.org which makes her efforts available to all of us (published with permission). Table 16.3 lists some recommended websites but you will find others as you search. The only way to find good material is to browse. Some useful search terms which can be used in Google are "medical education", "bedside teaching", "lecturing", "small-group teaching," "adult learning", and "faculty development". If you use the search string, "faculty development" in medical education, you will find websites which are devoted to medical educators. A useful, free online site is the Best Evidence Medical Education (BEME) www.bemecollaboration.org/ (accessed 8/18/07). Their site states:

> The BEME Collaboration is a group of individuals or institutions who are committed to the promotion of BEME through:
> - the dissemination of information which allows medical teachers, institutions and all concerned with medical education to make decisions on the basis of the best evidence available;
> - the production of appropriate systematic reviews of medical education which reflect the best evidence available and meet the needs of the user;
> - the creation of a culture of best evidence medical education amongst individual teachers, institutions and national bodies.

**Table 16.3** Websites containing faculty development information and medical education resources.

| Name of organization/individuals | Value of Website | Address |
| --- | --- | --- |
| Mary Jo Wagner and Sam Luber | List of medical education and faculty development websites | www.emergencymeducation.org |
| Professional and Organizational Network for Higher Education | Supports faculty teaching in higher education. Requires a yearly membership fee | www.podnetwork.org |
| ACGME | Has a huge amount of information on teaching residents. Lists the residency review requirements for emergency medicine | http://www.acgme.org/acWebsite/RRC |
| AAMC | Lists (1) organizations involved in medical education, (2) has the MedEdPortal which is a site which will peer review submitted educational materials and (3) other resources for both faculty and medical students | http://www.aamc.org/meded/start.htm |
| AAMC | This is another AAMC website with "Comprehensive Information for Medical Faculty" on a variety of topics | http://www.aamc.org/members/facultydev |
| BEME | Disseminates information, publishes systematic reviews, and creates a culture of "best evidence in medical education" | www.bemecollaboration.org |

*Continued*

| Name of organization/individuals | Value of Website | Address |
|---|---|---|
| AERA | Contains information of interest to educators and publishes the journal Educational Researcher. Site has a fee for access | http://www.aera.net |
| ERIC sponsored by the U.S. Department of Education, Institute of Education Sciences | Provides free access to over 1.2 million records of journal articles and other education-related materials | http://www.eric.ed.gov/ |
| SAEM Simulation Interest Group | Many educational materials compiled by emergency physicians. Some materials only accessible to interest group members | http://www.emedu.org/sim/ |

The above resources pertain largely to medical education and adult learning. This does not begin to tap into educational and psychological journals and sites which can have useful information. The American Educational Research Association (AERA) http://www. aera.net/ (paid membership required) has a great deal of information and the society publishes the journal *Educational Researcher* which has articles on general education. Frequently you can access this journal for free from your university. The Educational Resources Information Center (ERIC) http://www.eric.ed.gov/ is a free site, sponsored by the U.S. Department of Education, Institute of Education Sciences, which has a wealth of information, providing free access to over 1.2 million records of journal articles and other education-related materials. Unfortunately, much of it is not peer-reviewed and it is not as well indexed as Medline, so "buyer beware" with some of the material being very good. As your interest in certain topics within medical education grows, accessing this literature and these sites may be very useful.

Many emergency medicine faculty are working in the frontiers of simulation, both within their departments and in their medical schools, and have generously placed a lot of the materials they have developed online.

A librarian can be very helpful in performing searches of both written materials and online resources. They are eager to help physicians and will often teach you many of their techniques as well as performing requested searches.

## Formal faculty development programs

There are many formal faculty development programs. They can be found in professional societies, university and medical school settings, libraries, and in some community hospitals. A group from BEME-reviewed published literature on faculty development programs in medical education from 1980 to 2002 for effects on participants. http://www.bemecollaboration.org/beme/files/ BEME%20Guide%20no%208/BEME%20Review%20Text.pdf Accessed 8/31/07 [6]. The articles showed that the majority of programs focused on practicing clinicians and, in general, did have a positive effect. Participants were highly satisfied. There was gain in knowledge, skills, and attitudes, and positive self-reported or observed changes in teaching behaviors. Table 16.4 lists the key features of effective faculty development programs and can be used when looking for quality programs.

The first programs for discussion are those which are short in length, known personally to the author, or have been recommended by other emergency physicians. Many of these offerings are superb in quality (Table 16.5). The table does not include courses offered by an individual hospital or university.

**Table 16.4** Characteristics of successful faculty development programs.

Use of experiential learning

Provision of feedback

Effective peer and colleague relationships

Well-designed interventions following good principles of instruction

Multiple methods of teaching and learning used

Longer programs (more than 1–2 days) seemed to be more effective

**Table 16.5** Faculty development courses of emergency medicine organizations.

| Organization | Name of programme and content | Contact information |
| --- | --- | --- |
| CORD | Academic Assembly | http:///www.cord.org |
| SAEM | Annual Meeting | http://www.saem.org |
| EMF and ACEP | Emergency Medicine Teaching Fellowship | http://www.acep.org |
| ACEP | Advanced Teaching Fellowship | http://www.acep.org |
| ACEP | Emergency Medicine Basic Research Skills (EMBRS) | http://www.acep.org |
| SAEM EBM Interest Group IG | Evidence Based Emergency Medicine Workshop | http://ebem.org/ brochure.html |
| CAEP | ED STAT! | http://www.caep.ca |

The CORD sponsors an annual spring meeting, The Academic Assembly, which is devoted to the education of faculty though out their academic careers. The program has a variety of offerings, divided into tracks for junior or senior faculty, new program directors, and residency coordinators. While content varies somewhat from year to year, the program always includes discussions on teaching from emergency medicine physicians who are nationally recognized for their skills in this area. The meeting has increased in length but currently the program for junior faculty is 2.5 days in length and that targeted at senior faculty is 1.5 days. It is important to note that participants are encouraged to attend any topics they are interested in learning about rather than rigidly choosing one track. Information concerning this program can be found on the CORD website, http://www.cordem.org/.

The SAEM puts on an annual meeting which has presentations of interest to educators and researchers, as well as providing a forum for oral and poster presentations of research and educational materials and methods. It also sponsors interest groups such as the EBM and simulation interest groups which submit educational proposals for presentation at the meeting.

The ACEP and the Emergency Medicine Foundation sponsor the EMF/ACEP Teaching Fellowship. This is a 12 day course spread over 2 weeks, one in the fall and one in the spring. Didactic and bedside teaching, curriculum design, career and leadership development, and evaluation are all taught. Participants complete a scholarly project which is presented in the second week. One of the most valuable portions is "micro teaching" by participants when they are videotaped to improve their teaching. There is also an Advanced Teaching Fellowship sponsored by ACEP which is a 2.5 day course. While the content varies from year to year, subjects have included bedside teaching, using multimedia for teaching, successful lecturing, and finding educational resources. The ACEP sponsors a 12 day program, divided into two sessions, Emergency Medicine Basic Research Skills (EMBRS) which is targeted at junior faculty and other emergency physicians interested in gaining a basic understanding of how to perform research.

Members of the SAEM EBM Interest Group have made it their mission to teach physicians to utilize the principles of EBM in their daily practices and teach the principles to residents and medical students. They give courses at professional meetings and present a 2 day course at the New York Academy of Medicine.

ED STAT! (Emergency Department Strategies for Teaching any Time) is sponsored by the Canadian Association of Emergency Physicians (CAEP) and focuses on various aspects of teaching. It is modular in concept and can be adapted to various settings (0.5 to 2 days). Faculty will come to a department to teach or individual doctors can attend a session in Canada. Information can be found by going to the CAEP web site, www.caep.ca.

The American Association of Medical College (AAMC) sponsors the Medical Education Research Certification program which is a series of 6 workshops, each 3 hours in length, that teach educators to conduct educational research. The Harvard Macy Institute conducts a Program for Physician–Educators which focuses most directly on the educational issues of how to design and implement new curricula and pedagogical reforms or assessment methods within a course or a department. Stanford University offers a teaching fellowship which is highly regarded and concentrates on teaching.

Many universities offer courses on education but there are very few degreed medical education programs. For those wanting advanced degrees in education the possibilities include a master's degree, doctoral degree, and an education specialist degree. In 2005 Cohen and colleagues updated formal programs which offered master's degrees in medical education [7]. They identified 21 programs offered by universities, six located in the U.S. Their article is of value for contact information, duration, and delivery format.

It is important to remember that physicians interested in medical education may enroll in related programs such as instructional technology or adult education. Physicians may begin searching for programs by contacting the faculty development offices at their university and medical school. The College of Education in their university may offer related programs which will meet their educational goals and needs.

## Promotion

Many universities and medical schools are now restructuring their promotion guidelines to allow clinicians to be promoted on the basis of a combination of teaching, service, and scholarly activities, rather than only demanding large portfolios in research [4]. It is imperative that faculty understand the promotion and tenure guidelines at their institution since universities differ widely in how they interpret the meaning of scholarly activity as well as the weight they place on teaching, service, and scholarship when reviewing a candidate's application for promotion. In any event, it is necessary to carefully document teaching and scholarly activities. The use of an educator's portfolio is a tool that allows this documentation in a clear and detailed manner [8]. A table which documents the type of teaching performed with dates, the learners taught, the materials produced to aid in teaching, and finally the evaluation of teaching is a clear and concise method to demonstrate productivity and excellence. Listing honors acquired for excellence in teaching is also extremely helpful. The number of universities and medical schools requiring an educator's portfolio as part of the promotion documentation is increasing [9].

## Pitfalls

There are a number of potential pitfalls in academics. (1) Working in a medical school or university which highly values bench and clinical research if you are interested primarily in teaching and performing a variety of scholarly activities including some educational research. This can be avoided by looking at the promotion and tenure guidelines of the institution at the time of recruitment, talking to a number of faculty in various departments, and looking to see how many emergency medicine physicians have been promoted to associate or full professor. (2) Staying in a department which demands a heavy clinical commitment and does not provide any protected time for academics. (3) Expecting a large amount of protected time for anticipated projects you wish to do. The Chair has a finite number of resources and may not be able to provide protected time until you have made some academic contributions and carved out a niche for yourself. (4) Not finding a mentor who can help you perform research, become known in the academic community, and give you guidance for your career path. (5) Expecting promotion with few or no publications. Publishing in peer-reviewed journals is a requirement of almost all academic institutions and promotion committees wish to see evidence of expertise in your chosen area as proven by multiple publications on a particular topic.

## Conclusion

Becoming an expert in teaching requires the same thoughtful preparation and knowledge that any successful career demands. Expert medical teachers need content knowledge of medicine, knowledge about adult learning, and the desire to share what they know with others. Faculty development courses are valuable to help educators improve their teaching. Teaching, scholarly activities, and service must be well documented if educators are to succeed in the promotion process.

### Summary points

Do

Before taking a position:
1. Read the promotion and tenure guidelines of the institution, understand faculty tracks if present and requirements for promotion in the track in which you will be placed.
2. Find out if tenure is required by the institutions.
3. Find out the rank of emergency department faculty and length of time to promotion.
4. Find out if you will have a title, protected time, and what faculty track you will be placed on.
5. Talk to faculty about their protected time, if they have been able to find mentors in the institution and if they are given opportunity to teach and engage in scholarly activity.

Once you have a position:
1. Read the promotion and tenure guidelines of the institution, understand faculty tracks if present and requirements for promotion in the track in which you are placed.
2. Join emergency medicine professional societies involved in teaching and become active by joining committees or interest groups.
3. Network with your colleagues both in your institution and the societies you join.
4. Attend the Academic Assembly and consider taking the EMF/ ACEP Teaching Fellowship.
5. Read articles on teaching, watch the teaching style of others, and learn from evaluations of your teaching. Be prepared to change for improvement.
6. Explore your institution for faculty development programs.
7. Put together short- and long-term goals and ask to discuss them during your evaluation by the Chair. Be prepared to demonstrate what you have accomplished.
8. Begin an Educator's Portfolio.
9. Find a mentor(s).

10. Publish either clinical or educational research. (Take a course on manuscript preparation and professional writing, read texts on how to write professionally if you are uncomfortable with writing.)
11. If you agree to work on a project meet deadlines.
12. Be a team player.
13. Talk to the Chair and learn how you can help advance the mission and needs of the department.

Don't

1. Expect to have a large amount of protected time at the beginning of your career.
2. Expect to be given a title with a great deal of responsibility before you have spent time in the department and demonstrated your capabilities.
3. Promise to work on projects and then not fulfill obligations and meet deadlines.
4. Stay in a department if you are not given credit for your work or the clinical duty expectations make it impossible to perform scholarly activity.
5. Expect to only work on your goals; the department has needs that faculty must meet.

## References

1. The Professional and Organizational Network for Higher Education. *Faculty Development Definitions,* 2007.
2. Gruppen LD, *et al.* Educational fellowship programs: Common themes and overarching issues. *Acad Med* 2006; 81(11): 990–994.
3. Boyer E. *Scholarship Reconsidered: Priorities of the Professoriate.* Foundation for the Advancement of Teaching, Princeton, NJ, 1990.
4. Bunton SA, Mallon WT. The continued evolution of faculty appointment and tenure policies at U.S. medical schools. *Acad Med* 2007; 82(3): 281–289.
5. Wilkerson L, Irby DM. Strategies for improving teaching practices: A comprehensive approach to faculty development. *Acad Med* 1998; 73(4): 387–396.
6. Steinert Y, *et al. A Systematic Review of Faculty Development Initiatives Designed to Improve Teaching Effectiveness in Medical Education* BEME, 2002 Guide No 8.
7. Cohen R, *et al.* An update on master's degrees in medical education. *Med Teach* 2005; 27(8): 686–692.
8. Kuhn GJ. Faculty development: The educator's portfolio: Its preparation, uses, and value in academic medicine. *Acad Emerg Med* 2004; 11(3): 307–311.

9. Simpson D, *et al.* Documentation systems for educators seeking academic promotion in U.S. medical schools. *Acad Med* 2004; 79(8): 783–790.

## Recommended reading

Boyer E. *Scholarship Reconsidered: Priorities of the Professoriate.* Foundation for the Advancement of Teaching, Princeton, NJ, 1990.

Bunton SA, Mallon WT. The continued evolution of faculty appointment and tenure policies at U.S. medical schools. *Acad Med* 2007; 82(3): 281–289.

Ericsson KA. Deliberate practice and the acquisition and maintenance of expert performance in medicine and related domains. *Acad Med* 2004; 79(10 Suppl): S70–S81.

Gruppen LD, Simpson D, *et al.* Educational fellowship programs: Common themes and overarching issues. *Acad Med* 2006; 81(11): 990–994.

Hamilton GC, Brown JE. Faculty development: What is faculty development?" *Acad Emerg Med* 2003; 10(12): 1334–1336.

Hammoud M, Gruppen L, *et al.* To the Point: reviews in medical education online computer assisted instruction materials. *Am J Obstet Gynecol* 2006; 194(4): 1064–1069.

Huth EJ. *How to Write and Publish Papers in the Medical Sciences.* Williams and Wilkins, Baltimore, 1990.

King LS. *Why not Say it Clearly: A Guide to Expository Writing.* Little Brown, Boston, 1991.

Kuhn GJ. Faculty development: The educator's portfolio: Its preparation, uses, and value in academic medicine. *Acad Emerg Med* 2004; 11(3): 307–311.

Lujan HL, DiCarlo SE. Too much teaching, not enough learning: What is the solution? *Adv Physiol Educ* 2006; 30(1): 17–22.

Norman, G. *International Handbook of Research in Medical Education.* International Handbooks of Education, Kluwe Academic Publishers, Dordrecht/Boston, London, 1999.

Ramani S, Gruppen L. *et al.* Twelve tips for developing effective mentors. *Med Teach* 2006; 28(5): 404–408.

Simpson D, Hafler J, *et al.* Documentation systems for educators seeking academic promotion in U.S. medical schools. *Acad Med* 2004; 79(8): 783–790.

**SECTION 5**
# Teaching Techniques and Strategies

# CHAPTER 17

# Strategies for effective clinical emergency department teaching

*Glen Bandiera[1], Shirley Lee[2]*
[1]*University of Toronto; St. Michael's Hospital, Toronto, ON, Canada*
[2]*Schwartz/Reisman Emergency Centre, Faculty of Medicine, University of Toronto; Mount Sinai Hospital, Toronto, ON, Canada*

## Introduction

For emergency physicians (EPs) working in a busy, unpredictable, and physically constrained environment, the only practical teaching strategies are those that are both efficient and effective [1–4]. Few education studies have addressed the unique Emergency Department (ED) context; and adapting general ambulatory care models to the ED requires insight, thought, and concerted effort [5–7]. This chapter describes two models for ED teaching – a popular ambulatory model that can be adapted to the ED and another derived specifically for ED teaching based on primary ED education research.

## Strategies versus traits

Many studies of effective teachers address traits, rather than behaviors [5, 6]. Success as a teacher, however, depends on how these personal traits actually manifest in practice. The literature identifies the following positive traits of effective teachers: approachability, enthusiasm, content expertise, good communication skills, sensitivity to different supervisory needs, and willingness to take the time to teach [5, 8, 9]. But how does one use content expertise

*Practical Teaching in Emergency Medicine*, 1st edition. Edited by R Rogers, A Mattu, M Winters & J Martinez. ©2009 Blackwell Publishing, ISBN: 9781405176224

to get the most out of a teaching point? And how exactly does one take the time to teach when, seemingly, there is barely time for patient care? Good ED teachers recognize which of their strengths are conducive to effective teaching and actively adapt teaching strategies to both their environment and circumstances. The following sections detail a number of these strategies for ED teaching and describe how they can be easily implemented using either of two integrative models.

## Models to guide ED teaching

Expert teachers and learners agree on what behaviors make for good teachers [4, 10]. Just as there is an approach to acute trauma resuscitation or the work-up of patients with dizziness, there is an approach to a teaching encounter. One popular approach to ambulatory teaching, Nehrer's microskills [7], was developed in the clinic environment. The five steps have some applicability to the ED and are briefly described in the next paragraphs. A second model, described by the acronym "E.D.S.T.A.T" (Figure 17.1), was based on primary ED research and is presented in detail in the remainder of the chapter. There is significant overlap between the models and each will appeal to different teachers' perspectives. Specific strategies to implement the steps in both models will be described using examples from the literature, our own research, and our experiences. Strategies specific to microskills are presented along with the discussion of Nehrer's model; strategies applicable to both models and those specific to E.D.S.T.A.T. are presented with that model.

The first microskill, "Get a commitment," involves encouraging the learner to make a decision based on the information they have gathered. The commitment can relate to any aspect of the

Expectations
Diagnose the learner

Setup
Teach
Assess and give feedback
Teacher always (role model)

**Figure 17.1** The ED STAT teaching model.

physician–patient interaction from differential diagnosis through to investigations and on to disposition decisions. The ED is an ideal environment to implement this step given the high volume and diversity of patients seen. The more senior the learner, the more sophisticated the level of commitment can be. Success in this step requires a sound learning environment in which a learner can feel both empowered and safe to make decisions. The second step, "probe for supporting evidence," involves asking the learner why they have made the decision they did. This exercise creates a level of meta-cognition that allows the learner to gain insights into why they make the decisions they do and provide the teacher with evidence about the learner's diagnostic reasoning. In the ED, learners are constantly faced with uncertainty and value the good teachers who know what key elements in a presentation guide their decision making and take the opportunity to impart this experience to learners. "Teach general rules" allows learners to apply lessons to a breadth of circumstances. A typical ED example might be "sudden onset pain is a vascular catastrophe until proven otherwise." The last two microskills "reinforce what was done right" and "correct mistakes" relate to feedback. Good ED teachers provide feedback to learners that it is contextual, frequent, and related to specific actions rather than to characteristics. They do not wait until the end of a rotation or even a shift to provide feedback and avoid the temptation to limit feedback to generalities as exemplified by comments such as "great job today, keep it up!"

The E.D.S.T.A.T. model has two phases. The first involves setting Expectations (E) and Diagnosing the learner (D). These critical steps taken when a teacher first interacts with a learner underpin both efficiency and effectiveness. When done well, the remainder of the strategies is much more easily implemented. The second phase frames each individual teaching encounter, and involves a Setup (S), a specific Teaching point or principle (T), Assessment or feedback (A), and role modeling through demonstration and clinical practice: the realization that one is a Teacher always (T).

## When you first encounter a learner: E and D

### Expectations
Efficient teachers invest small amounts of time getting to know learners, establishing early on what their educational needs are. Only then can they choose high-impact material that will be

remembered by learners for its utility and relevance. Learners' perceptions of the amount and quality of teaching is influenced positively by the relevance of the material to them and the perceived amount of effort the teacher spent adapting to the learner's needs. Discussing expectations takes about 5–10 minutes at the beginning of a shift. Good teachers view this as time well spent, allowing for greater efficiencies later. Learners appreciate the interest and the teacher can then cleverly demonstrate this interest when later they direct the learner to a specific patient problem the learner had identified as an educational need, or review a key differential diagnosis the learner had previously mentioned as challenging for them.

Learners do not always know what is best for them. Teachers should play an active role in objective setting. Setting expectations includes consideration of objectives set by learners and their program, specific patients of interest to the learner, and points along the patient interview-synthesis-investigation-management spectrum where the learner typically encounters difficulty. Questions such as "What do you want to learn/see today" or "What learning objectives do you have?" often fail to elicit objective responses from trainees who are eager to appear interested in everything. Examples such as "What do you normally find challenging/interesting/difficult?," "What was on your wish list that you have yet to see?," "What feedback have you been given about areas to work on?," "What would you like me to provide feedback on today?," or "What types of patients should I be on the lookout for today that you would like to see?" may be more likely to elicit tangible objectives. Learners should be reassured that setting expectations is in their best interest: "how will we know if we've accomplished any learning today?" or "I can't involve you in the high-yield cases if I don't know what those are!" It may be helpful to allow time to think about expectations by revisiting the questions part way through the shift or forewarning learners about the need to define objectives in an orientation session or package prior to the rotation. Expectations can evolve as a teacher and learner each become familiar with what the other has to offer. For example, as a learner masters certain content areas, new objectives will need to be developed. Alternatively, experience in the ED may uncover unexpected areas of need. Learners should be exposed to specific patients and problems that they may not see elsewhere. EDs with specific mandates such as trauma, inner-city health, or community-based practice should encourage learners to take advantage of these.

Teachers with specific interests should make these known to the learner and devise objectives around these. For example, an EP with an interest in toxicology, trauma, or clinical epidemiology might be a huge opportunity for a learner.

Expectations should take on more breadth for senior learners. Teaching, administrative issues, managerial skills, or risk management/quality improvement activities are fair objectives. With senior learners there is often more difficulty establishing the appropriate amount of supervision. Questions such as "How would you like me to be involved today?," "Should we share the teaching?," "What logistical issues frustrate you?," or "What cases are you comfortable handling on your own?" often elicit helpful responses.

Some learners are self-directed and wish to think through problems on their own using notes or web-based resources; others prefer to optimize their time with an "expert" to discuss an approach. Some respond well to guiding questions while others see these as a frustrating "read my mind" challenge. Visual learners benefit more from reading than from a lecture on a topic. Learners frequently lack the insight required to articulate these nuances at first and teachers may need to revise their approach over time based on their experience. Again, asking these types of questions is not futile: it serves to demonstrate your interest in the learner and highlight to them the need for some self-insight.

Teachers should disclose their own teaching habits. Learners are frustrated when different teachers have different expectations and they are constantly trying to "guess" what the teacher wants. Discussing a preference clearly sends the message that the teacher understands the students' perspective. Subsequent teaching will be more efficient because the learner can adapt their presentations to the teacher's expectations. For example, do you like the learner to summarize the history, examination, differential diagnosis, and management plan or do you prefer that the learner state up front what they think is going on and then probe their rationale through questioning? Do you like learners to review all patients prior to ordering investigations or are you comfortable with them ordering basic investigations on their own? How many patients should they have "on the go" before coming to review them? The answers to these questions will vary depending on learner level and your comfort with them.

Some learners benefit from stringent guidelines. Setting time limits on patient interactions, breaks and departures from the department are important, especially for learners who are not as organized and for those unfamiliar with the ED. Learners often have difficulty understanding that ED assessments can be focused and would benefit from some clarity on your expectations regarding patient flow. Medical students and junior residents should likely focus more on quality care for a fewer number of patients and leave streamlining and cognitive short cuts to more senior residents.

## Diagnosing the learner

Learners' strengths and limitations, the teacher's experience with the learner, and in some cases knowledge about the learner's prior performance all inform a teacher's impression or "diagnosis" of the learner. This represents recognition of what cognitive and behavioral level the learner is at and a decision on a course of action to advance this level. At this stage obvious areas of concern or deficiencies should be noted by the teacher, and any significant concerning behaviors identified. The teacher can then make a decision about how they will interact with the learner, what they will teach, and what degree of autonomy they will provide.

For example, learners who are slow to decide on a disposition or are overly conservative may be risk averse. These learners should be encouraged to make decisions and commit to a course of action within the security of a supervised environment. Some learners will be "minimizers" and others "worriers." Teachers should adapt their vigilance accordingly. Learners may avoid certain patients because they have deficiencies in their patient care skill set. They should be encouraged to face their limitations head-on with additional guidance or tools from the teacher. Some learners have specific deficits in core competencies such as diagnostic reasoning, communication skills, teamwork ability, resource management, professionalism, or critical appraisal. Astute teachers will be vigilant for these deficits and will tailor their approach to help address these through teaching and feedback. Learners should be aware and ideally agree that these will be areas of focus. Clearly, teachers who are effective at discussing expectations will have the least difficulty with learner diagnosis.

## For each teaching encounter: STAT

### Setup
Learners often require sensitization to learning points or guidance around the approach to a patient problem. This can be accomplished

with a brief set up discussion. Careful setup will teach the learner about what is important in a given presentation, provide specific guidelines around a patient encounter, and alert them to teaching that will follow. For rudimentary or familiar presentations, many learners will appropriately engage patients on their own with little or no setup.

Setup may include medical decision making: "this patient is here with right upper quadrant abdominal pain – what are the five most important diagnoses you are going to consider?," or "this patient is here with chest pain – I want you to bring the ECG to me within 5 minutes if it is anything but normal – reducing time to acute MI treatment is one of the biggest impacts we can make in emergency medicine" or "this patient seems to have multiple complaints – your job is to identify the principle complaint, the chronic problems, and if any of them seem dangerous – then be clear with the patient which we will and which we won't be able to address today."

In some cases, feedback provided for one case will set up the next. For example, if a student requires an inordinately long time to assess a straightforward ankle inversion, a teacher might use feedback about this to set up the next case: "I expect you to complete the history and examination in less than 15 minutes – if it seems it will take longer, I want you to come and tell me and we'll try and figure out why." If the student has a habit of this type of difficulty, this could have been identified during discussions of expectations, and would inform the teacher's diagnosis of the learner. Consistency through all phases of the teaching model can lead to very satisfying improvements in learner performance.

Some set up issues may pertain to department logistics: "our ultrasound department closes in 30 minutes – decide in the next 10 minutes if you think this patient will require an ultrasound – that's a patient flow tip I picked up a few years ago!" Still others may relate to key resources: "this pocket card is a clinical decision rule that I use for patients like this. Go see the patient, then have a look at it – your job is to tell me if you think they satisfy the components of the rule." Sensitize the learner to some of these efficiency measures by framing them as learning or practice "tips."

## Teach a focused teaching point

Excellent teachers do not necessarily teach the most. Rather, they teach high-yield material, relate it specifically to an individual learner, and make learning interactive and fun. Selecting an appropriate teaching point is an art. Good teaching points are (1) relevant to the learner (based on expectations, the learner's diagnosis, and possibly an appropriate setup), (2) contextual (learned in the course of patient care), (3) linked to previous knowledge (from past encounters with the learner and knowledge of their previous experiences), and (4) clearly identified as grounded in evidence, general opinion, or the teacher's own experience. Thankfully, learners do not expect long, thorough reviews of topics in the ED. They appreciate helpful guidance around patient care, "rules of thumb," useful resources, correction of inaccuracies or deficiencies in their knowledge base, and useful approaches to problems [11]. Many good teaching points will pertain to nonclinical issues such as good teaching practice, patient flow, or interprofessional relations.

Good teachers actively seek teaching opportunities. They listen to conversations learners have with each other and other health professionals. They read what learners chart and seek out interesting lab and imaging results. They summon all learners in the department for a brief teaching encounter around a great case, modified to each learner's level. Good teachers have a repository of resources that they use to support a teaching point or address a learner's declared learning need. Examples might include a digital image library, file of interesting EKGs or lab results, or favorite websites and practice guidelines. For senior residents, involving them in administrative decisions, diverting nurses' queries to them, and having triage personnel notify them first about trauma or resuscitation cases are all important opportunities.

Learners like to be challenged in a safe teaching environment. Success depends directly on proper learner diagnosis and preparing them for the challenge through the setting of proper expectations. Rather than focusing on what learners already know or what they can easily read in a textbook, good teachers promote active learning in three key ways. First, they quickly push learners to the limit of their knowledge and take them to the next step but rarely beyond. Asking for innovative differentials is a good way to do this: "list six extraperitoneal causes of abdominal pain," "what seven immediately life-threatening thoracic injuries must be sought in the primary survey of a trauma patient?" Good teachers expand on a case: "okay, it sounds like you know what to do with this patient, but how would that change if she were pregnant?," or "do you know what patient population that decision rule was derived and validated in?"

Learners appreciate flexibility in the approach to patients. It is essential that learners be forced to make decisions and as long as their proposal is safe, it is sometimes useful to allow them to carry out their plan even if it is not the teacher's first choice of actions. The learner can then adapt their approach through an iterative process by seeing the consequences of their decisions. At the very least learners should be forced to make a commitment and justify their opinion before the teacher explains why a different course of action should be taken.

Effective teachers have strategies for busy times. They acknowledge that detailed teaching will be replaced with more concise case-based teaching focused on learner needs. For example, if EKGs or radiographs have been identified as an area of concern, then teaching can focus on any EKG or imaging studies completed. Rather than teaching the approach to decreased level of consciousness for 30–45 minutes, teachers can focus on lab results such as acid–base "rules" or a differential for elevated anion gap. The learner can then be referred to a textbook or website for an overall algorithm. There can be a "theme of the day" such as the differential diagnosis of headache. In available moments, the learner can be prompted for another addition to their list and the teacher can commit to discussing the pertinent physical findings or investigations for every new item the learner adds. Finishing off the list can then become homework or a topic of discussion after the shift. Likewise, if a learner has difficulty deciding upon investigations but has decent assessment skills, the teacher can quickly satisfy themselves that the story is adequate (either by some brief questions to the learner or going in to see the patient themselves with the learner in tow) then focus teaching on investigations. For example, it would be more useful to focus on the limitations of ultrasound in diagnosing appendicitis than on the embryology of gut rotation and why the appendix is in the right lower quadrant. For a medical student an introductory line might be, "walk me through how you examined the abdomen – I've got a couple of tricks you may find useful then I'll tell you how I investigate these problems," whereas for a senior resident the focus may be "I've quickly talked to the patient you saw and I agree it sounds like it might be a pulmonary embolism, what do you know about the sensitivity of CT in the diagnosis?" Efficient teachers multitask by "teaching and doing" such as by "talking through" procedures for the benefit of learners.

Good teaching points can be overlooked. Simply telling a learner that the Ottawa Ankle Rule exists and where to find it is a useful 30-second teaching point. Going through the rule and its application is quite another, taking perhaps 5 or 10 minutes. Good teachers will recognize the difference between these two and adapt their approach to the time available. Another quick example for the student who has difficulty organizing a differential is to provide a mnemonic that they can use for all subsequent cases and insist they use it.

Finally, many excellent teachers make use of teaching scripts, described by Irby [11]. Teaching scripts are discrete packages of information that a teacher keeps in the back of their mind for popular scenarios that arise. Typically, the script will be based on the teacher's previous experience with learners at a similar level and focus on common areas of misconception or difficulty. The beauty of teaching scripts is that they are brief, targeted to common areas of need, and easy to carry out because the teacher is familiar with them. They can be delivered with minimal preparation.

## Assess and give feedback

While feedback is detailed in another chapter, it is important to note that good teachers provide both ongoing and summative feedback to learners. Feedback given in the course of case review can be used to set up future cases: "the most important thing you write in the chart is the discharge instructions. Please be specific about what you tell patients when they leave – I'll be looking for this in the next few charts you do." There is no better time to provide feedback about an incident than shortly after it has occurred, assuming the learner is receptive. The rare situation may arise when a particularly stressful or negative event has occurred when feedback should be deferred. It is important that learners be provided with guidance as they progress through the shift or at the very least a summary of feedback including specific references to important incidents, both good and bad, that occurred that day. The use of shift feedback cards is a good way to both stimulate and document feedback sessions.

## Teacher always: the role of role modeling

Much of the learning that occurs in the ED is implicit – learners observe what teachers say and do. Learners are frustrated when teachers do something they themselves advised against, or omit an action that they recently told the learner was necessary. It is thus important that teachers hold themselves to a high standard and display the behaviors and professionalism they expect from students. Teachers should acknowledge when something is their opinion and not an unequivocal truth. Learners will likely have seen a different approach in the recent past and be confused about contradictions in practice.

Learners must be skilled at identifying their limits. Teachers should also acknowledge when they do not know factual material or require additional expertise to manage a patient. This is seen by good teachers as an opportunity to team up with the learner to solve the problem: "you look here and I'll look there and we'll compare notes." This can also be turned into a homework assignment: "you look this up and see what you find – I'll do that same and we'll talk about it when we next meet." Teachers should demonstrate appropriate collaborative behavior with other health professions and physician colleagues and acknowledge when circumstances lead to suboptimal interactions on busy or frustrating days. Teachers should demonstrate to learners where their own learning opportunities arise: "I learned something today…" or "I'll definitely do that differently next time!"

## Summary

There are multiple strategies described here to help carry out effective ED teaching, tied together by the microskills or E.D.S.T.A.T. models. Setting expectations and diagnosing the learner establish rapport and help develop an effective, efficient learning plan. Most teaching encounters should include a setup, selection of a key teaching point, assessment, and feedback. Finally, teachers should do what they say and say what they do – they are always teaching through role modeling. It is not necessary to change all teaching behaviors at once – teaching can improve even with some incremental positive changes. Remember that learners benefit most from teachers who have the learners' best interests in mind, are proactive, and are willing to make changes in how they do things for better learning and clinical care.

**Summary points**

1. Be clear about your expectations and discuss how you like to review cases with the learner.
2. Form a "diagnosis" of the learner's needs, strengths, and liabilities based on your observations and discussions with the learner.
3. Set up each shift and patient interaction so the learner knows what to focus on.
4. Focus teaching around key points and direct learners towards reference materials for more comprehensive review.
5. Feedback, both positive and negative, is best given frequently and in the context of individual patient care.
6. Recognize the teacher's obligations as a role model – make sure you embody what you teach.

# References

1. Atzema C, Bandiera G, Schull MJ. Emergency department crowding: the effect on resident education. *Ann Emerg Med* 2005; 45: 276–281.
2. Chisholm CD, Collison E, Nelson D, Cornell W. Emergency department workplace interruptions: are emergency physicians "interrupt-driven" and "multitasking"? *Acad Emerg Med* 2000; 7: 1239–1243.
3. Penciner R. Clinical teaching in a busy emergency department: strategies for success. *Can J Emerg Med* 2002; 4(4): 286–288.
4. Bandiera G, Lee S, Tiberius R. Creating effective learning in today's emergency departments: how accomplished teachers get it done. *Acad Emerg Med* 2005; 45(3): 253–261.
5. Irby DM. Teaching and learning in ambulatory care settings: a thematic review of the literature. *Acad Med* 1995; 70: 898–931.
6. Heidenreich C, Lye P, Simpson D, Lourich M. The search for effective and efficient ambulatory teaching methods through the literature. *Pediatrics* 2000; 105 (Suppl 1): 231–237.
7. Neher JO, Gordon KC, Meyer B, Stevens N. A five-step "microskills" model of clinical teaching. *J Am Board Fam Pract* 1992; 5: 419–424.
8. Wolverton SE, Bosworth MF. A survey of resident perceptions of effective teaching behaviors. *Fam Med* 1985; 3: 106–108.
9. Wright SM, Kern DE, Koloder K, Howard DM, Brancati FL. Attributes of excellent attending-physician role models. *N Engl J Med* 1998; 339: 1986–1993.
10. Thurgur L, Bandiera G, Lee S, Tiberius R. What emergency medicine learners wish their teachers knew. *Acad Emerg Med* 2005; 12: 856–861.
11. Irby DM. What clinical teachers in medicine need to know. *Acad Med* 1994; 69: 333–342.

**CHAPTER 18**

# Pearls and pitfalls in teaching: what works, what doesn't?

*Brian Clyne, David G. Lindquist*
*Department of Emergency Medicine, The Warren Alpert Medical School of*
*Brown University, Providence, RI, USA*

## Introduction

The practice of medicine is built upon the time-honored tradition of passing knowledge from experienced clinicians to aspiring students at all levels. Regardless of one's specialty, level of experience, or practice setting, this custom is a defining feature of the profession. Nowhere is this process more evident than in emergency medicine (EM). High patient volumes, undifferentiated pathology, and direct supervision by experienced providers combine to create an environment rife with learning opportunities and the continuous exchange of ideas.

To write a chapter pointing out pitfalls without suggesting solutions would be akin to offering endless negative criticism to a student without offering ways to improve. Thus, while various pitfalls are highlighted, care is taken to offer alternative approaches. Naturally, many of these suggestions will reflect back on other chapters in this book, where various strategies for successful teaching are presented more extensively. Much of what is discussed here applies to bedside teaching, but many of the principles transfer readily to lecture preparation, the scripting of medical simulations, and the demonstration of procedures. The chapter that follows is

*Practical Teaching in Emergency Medicine*, 1st edition. Edited by R Rogers, A Mattu,
M Winters & J Martinez. ©2009 Blackwell Publishing, ISBN: 9781405176224

born primarily of experience, observation, and reflection. Our own missteps teaching EM have been a most powerful source for understanding what works and what doesn't.

Before engaging in any discussion of the teaching of EM, the importance of clinical competence must be recognized. Clinical excellence is a prerequisite for being a role model. You must have confidence in your clinical abilities to teach effectively and maintain credibility in your students' eyes.

Determining your own level of clinical competence requires that you assume the role of perpetual student assessing your strengths and weaknesses, seeking feedback, and taking the necessary steps to improve. Assuming this role will serve as a reminder that we are all students engaged in the medical tradition of passing along knowledge and experience.

## Teach for the right reasons

Teaching is hard, requires preparation time, and rarely comes naturally. If you are teaching primarily for personal gain (e.g. promotion), you may find its challenges intimidating. Your learners will quickly recognize your lack of enthusiasm for the task at hand, and your frustration at the workload will be apparent. Ideally, teaching is gratifying for you. To facilitate this, you should identify ways in which teaching enhances your own skills and judgment. Find opportunities to talk about what you know, or to learn more about a topic that you would like to master. Many people have an area about which they feel passionate, or at least to which they have a connection. Use that passion as a springboard to develop your teaching points. Channel your enthusiasm for the topic into your presentation. Teach as if you care. You may find that personal gain, once de-emphasized, comes more easily.

## Clarify expectations

One common pitfall for teachers is the failure to establish boundaries with one's students. This is especially true for junior faculty who, by virtue of their recent transition from residency, may regard senior residents more as peers than trainees. The crucial intellectual step for all faculty to take is to recognize how the responsibility for a trainee's education, and its direct impact on patient care, supersedes any desire to "be a pal."

A useful way to define your teaching role is to establish expectations for the learner. This avoids one of the classic pitfalls of clinical teaching, poorly communicated expectations. Well-defined goals, whether they are lecture objectives, how you prefer to hear patient presentations, or specific tasks you would like to see accomplished, will provide a constructive framework for teacher–student interactions and create a positive learning experience. When establishing the expectations, outline a few important areas on which they should focus. In EM, the goal is identifying acute problems, using focused history and physical examinations, sorting out the dangerous entities from the benign, and recognizing what is germane for the emergency department (ED). Offer guidance on what the EM priorities for a given patient. These clarified expectations make evaluation and feedback more straightforward, and provide that elusive overall sense of progress.

## Know what they need to learn

Whenever possible, determine the needs of your audience. Whether teaching at the bedside, lecturing to a crowd, or presenting to a small group, soliciting their goals and objectives will help you align them with your own. Assessing your learners' needs will allow you to target your instruction, establish your topic's relevance, and connect with your audience. You may consider showing how your topic will improve patient care, avoid lawsuits, increase efficiency, or as a last resort, pass the exam. Addressing your audience's goals and objectives is straightforward when groups have a shared level of expertise. Groups with varied levels of training demand a more thoughtful approach. The pitfall is teaching too narrowly. Aim too high, and your audience will fail to engage your topic. Aim for the least common denominator, and your audience will lose interest. A balanced presentation targets the objectives of your mid-range learners, offers pearls to your experts, yet remains accessible to all.

## Teach, don't taunt

We have all been subjected to that endless line of questioning that starts and ends with memorized medical facts, typically referred to as "pimping." Although falling out of favor, it deserves mention because it has been a common teaching method since the time of Sir William Osler. The recitation of mere information provides the learner no opportunity for "escape" or improvement. Pimping promotes a learned helplessness, whereby if the answer is not known, the student is left without recourse. At best, factual questioning establishes that the learner already knows whatever facts on which you quiz them. Using this method, the most you could hope to contribute to their education is a few more facts, often at the expense of the learner's self-esteem. If you are trying to gauge a learner's level of understanding, there may be a brief role for factual questioning, but it is otherwise a low-yield technique.

Instead, challenge the learner with questions that demand a problem-solving approach. Use nonthreatening questions that target students' understanding of broad concepts, rather than mundane facts. Regurgitating Ranson's Criteria is of little use if one does not understand the pathophysiology of pancreatitis. Focus your questions instead on the underlying mechanisms of pancreatitis. Students will ponder the processes and will transition easily to treatment considerations. They will have moved from the theoretical to the practical independently, experiencing the power of one to guide the other. Such critical thinking skills are relevant for emergency physicians, who make clinical decisions with limited information.

Emergency physicians are particularly adept at incorporating new teaching methods. The communication skills by which we connect with patients are precisely the ones which make an effective teacher. We make eye contact, listen, and provide explanations at the appropriate level. Use these same techniques to let your student feel that he/she has your full attention. Protect the encounter from interruption, listen attentively, paraphrase their comments, and address their questions thoughtfully.

## Activate your learners

Recognize that adults learn through action, experience, and reflection, rather than the passive absorption of information. Although lectures defy these basic principles, it must be acknowledged that a lecture format can be an effective way to convey information to a large group in a short time period. This one-way flow of ideas, from lecturer to audience, can be improved when the material is case-based, relevant to the audience's needs, and when the presentation allows for open discussion. Judiciously used, lectures can provide a basis from which other teaching methods can be implemented, including small group discussions, simulation exercises, or procedural skill training. These latter techniques are examples of more active learning that engage students, facilitate questions, and provide the opportunity for timely feedback.

Opportunities for active learning in the ED abound. Ideally, teaching is case-based, clinically relevant, protected from interruption, and consists of the exchange of ideas. Fortunately, sign-out rounds include all of these elements, in addition a receptive audience. This combination creates an extremely teachable moment. The physician leading rounds, can select teaching points based on the educational benefit to the team. The lead instructor should focus on key points and general guidelines, minimize factual questions, and ask questions of the group to establish a collaborative learning approach. Sign out gives trainees the opportunity to explain not just their management plans, but their decision-making process. This forces learners to employ critical thinking skills, review their patients' management, and take an active role in educating their peers.

Independent learning, such as researching a topic for a mini-lecture at the end of a shift, is another effective active learning strategy. Ideally, the topic stems from a clinical question that arose during the shift. Placing the student in a teaching role forces them to define the question and present the information clearly. There are many good structured case-based clinical teaching methods, described earlier in this book and elsewhere in the medical literature. Regardless of the method selected, their common value is the one-on-one exchange that occurs between teacher and student.

## A little autonomy goes a long way

One common pitfall in clinical teaching is the inability to extend control to your trainees. This may stem from a desire to maintain patient safety or departmental flow. As the shift gets busier, the temptation to take over patient care directly and have the student "learn by observation" becomes strong. The higher acuity a patient, and the less experienced the trainee, the harder it is to delegate decision-making responsibility. At every stage of training, provide greater responsibility and fewer limitations. Let your trainees know that when you ask "What do you want to do?" their response matters. Some trainees will continually defer to you. Guide them with your knowledge, experience, and the evidence

available, but resist the temptation to offer your opinion until they
have committed to their own plan. This forces them to consider
consequences, and eventually increases their comfort with the
decision-making role.

Relinquishing control can be a challenge, and clearly, patient
safety is foremost. But the medical student can be tasked with
deciding whether to order a complete blood count (CBC), the
intern whether a chest x-ray is needed to treat a pneumonia,
and the senior resident with the choice of noninvasive versus
endotracheal intubation. This graded approach can help you as the
teacher to become more comfortable with your trainees' growing
independence. In addition, the increased autonomy will force your
learner into a more active role.

## Keep it simple

Long lectures and comprehensive reviews are not only tedious, but
they are also impractical for the ED. Instead, keep discussions and
presentations focused on a specific problem, reinforcing your points
with relevant background information only. Avoid attempting to
convey too many concepts at once. This applies to lecture, bedside
teaching, simulation, and any other teaching venue. Select two or
three main points, avoid digressions, and provide the repetition that
promotes retention. The same principles apply when demonstrating
a procedure. Break it up into logical components (e.g. indications,
landmarks, site prep, execution, troubleshooting), pause for clarification and reinforcement, and allow time for questions.

## Practice safe learning

Belittle your learners for wrong answers or the sake of a laugh,
and you will firmly establish an audience that will not dare to
voice their opinions. A safe learning environment is paramount for
learners to venture beyond their comfort zone. If they fear humiliation, you will crimp their ability to think broadly, stand by their
reasoning, and make a commitment. Establish a climate where
learners feel comfortable expressing themselves by inviting their
opinions, encouraging their questions, and acknowledging your
own limitations. A nonthreatening working relationship provides
unforeseen benefits to patient care. A trainee may include information you had not considered, altering the patient's management.

Empowering trainees to voice their thoughts is consistent with the growing emphasis on teamwork training, communication, and their impact on patient safety.

## What are you thinking?

Conveying your thought process to your students and physicians-in-training is at the core of clinical teaching. Just as patients wish to know the reasons for their tests/treatments, so your students crave insight regarding your decisions. Elaborating on our thought process while caring for many patients is a constant challenge but it is the goal to which academic clinicians aspire.

One effective teaching method is to explain to the patient and the student simultaneously. This saves time, includes patients in the decision-making, and allows you to model the patient–physician interaction style you would like to impart. It is a powerful technique when you are uncertain as to the appropriate patient disposition, or sense resistance from the patient regarding your plan. When the student observes you summarize the case, outline the options, solicit the patient's and the family's input, and reach a consensus plan, then they will see a complete physician in action. They will see not only the medical decisions being made, but a model for how to address clinical, psychosocial, follow-up, and liability issues all in one brief encounter.

## Food for thought

Providing appropriate feedback may be the most difficult teaching task. Because most physicians feel uncomfortable offering it, they fall into the classic pitfalls of providing no feedback at all, or simply the vague reassurance that a trainee is "performing at a level appropriate for their training." This common criticism of medical education can be overcome not only with practice but also requires a constructive framework for giving objective feedback.

At baseline, there must be a professional culture of understanding. The teacher must recognize their responsibility for the student's improvement. Viewed in this light, feedback becomes an expectation, and a guide for professional development, not a judgment of character. Mature learners recognize this; those who become defensive upon receiving such critiques may benefit from having this dynamic pointed out.

Clarify at the outset the criteria by which the student will be judged. Set the expectations early. In this way, feedback becomes part of a discussion already begun, and feels less awkward.

To begin a feedback session, ask the student for a self-assessment. Often they will identify the same deficiencies you have, making the discussion easier. Keep the session on a professional level by referring to specific behaviors or actions that can be changed, and by using nonjudgmental, descriptive terms. Students will be more receptive to negative feedback if it is balanced by noting their areas of strength. Providing feedback in the appropriate setting is also important. The management phrase "Praise in public, criticize in private," applies here. End each session on a positive note, with concrete suggestions that the student can implement to improve. The weaker the trainee, the more specific behaviors you can list.

When giving feedback, do not overlook your strongest trainees. Although it may feel easier to evaluate them with a pat on the back, they are as deserving of guidance as their peers. Even the highest performers have room to improve.

## Summary

Despite its challenges, teaching EM can be intensely gratifying. The desire to share knowledge and expertise is a defining feature of our specialty. Our residencies are full of trainees eager to learn, and our responsibility to train them is enormous. We hope the pearls and pitfalls offered in this chapter will help you avoid the mistakes we have all made, and take advantage of the rich teaching environment in which we are privileged to practice.

|  | What works | What doesn't |
| --- | --- | --- |
| *Teach for the right reasons* | Teaching what you care about | Teaching for personal gain |
| *Clarify expectations* | Well-defined goals and objectives | Failing to establish roles |
| *Learn what they need to learn* | Assessing your learner's needs | Teaching too narrowly |
| *Teach, don't taunt* | Questions that foster problem-solving | Humiliation, sarcasm, and intimidation |

*Continued*

|  | What works | What doesn't |
| --- | --- | --- |
| *Activate your learners* | Engaging students, facilitating questions, providing feedback | Overuse of lecture format |
| *A little autonomy goes a long way* | Delegation of graded responsibility | Inability to relinquish control |
| *Keep it simple* | Problem-focused discussions | Information overload |
| *Practice safe learning* | Soliciting students' opinions and questions | Emphasizing the academic hierarchy |
| *What are you thinking?* | Explaining your thought process | Answers, not explanations |
| *Food for thought* | Timely, objective feedback | Personal character judgment |

# Index

academic setting, practicing in, 193–4

Accreditation Council for Graduate Medical Education (ACGME), 69, 114, 128, 200
core competencies, 131, 132
practice-based learning and improvement, 135–6
professionalism, 135
system-based practice, 132–5
Outcome Project, 131

active learner, 181

active learning, 39, 220, 229

adult learning, 3
educating adults, 7
in emergency department, 7
environment setting, 8–10
evaluation, 12–13
goals setting, 10–11
new materials, planning and implementing, 11–12
role model, 13–14
learning
as adult, 5–7
as child, 4
theories, 4

Advanced Teaching Fellowship, 199, 204

American Association of Emergency Medicine (AAEM), 198

American Association of Medical College (AAMC), 200, 205

American College of Emergency Physicians (ACEP), 198, 204

American Educational Research Association (AERA), 201, 202

andragogy, 5

*Annals of Emergency Medicine*, 75

"audience of one" technique, 174

balanced presentation, 227

barriers
to bedside teaching, 36–7
to enhance communication and professionalism, 88
to successful teachers, 164–5

bedside educator, 116, 119–21

bedside encounter, 36, 40

bedside questioning, 41–3

bedside teachers
characteristics of, 37–9

bedside teaching, in emergency department, 35, 56, 116–17
barriers, 36–7
bedside questioning, 41–3
effective bedside teachers, characteristics of, 37–9
experience versus explanation cycle, 39–41
feedback, providing, 43–5

beginning educator, 25

behavioral expectations, 44

behaviorism, 4

Best Evidence Medical Education (BEME), 199, 200

brainstorming, 185–6

breakout session, 182

briefing phase, 40

*British Medical Journal*, 199

"broad strokes", teaching, 148, 149

cadaver lab, 55–6, 57

Canadian Association of Emergency Physicians (CAEP), 203, 205

*Canadian Medical Association Journal,*
    199
case-based discussions, 117
case-based learning, 182
Centre for Evidence-Based
    Medicine, 75, 76
Centre for Health Evidence, 75
challenges of teaching in ED, 146,
    147
chaotic environment, effective
    teachers in, 136
childhood learning, 4
clerkship, 68, 109
clinical competence, 108, 226
clinical decision rules, 77, 82
clinical emergency department
    teaching, strategies for, 213
  expectations setting, 215–18
  feedback, to learners, 222
  focused teaching point, 219–22
  learner, diagnosing, 218
  role modeling, 223
  setup discussion, 218–19
  strategies versus traits, 213–14
  teaching models, 214–15
clinical encounter, 40
clinical teaching, 110–12
  paradigms, for EM faculty
    "educational nirvana",
      pursuing, 138
    effective teachers, in chaotic
      environment, 136
    knowledge retention,
      encouraging, 139–40
    multitasking, teaching, 141
    patients flow and acuity,
      approaches to, 136–8
    pattern recognition, 139
    resident errors, 141–2
    visual diagnosis, 139
clinicians as teachers, 194
closed questions, 185
cognitive learning theory, 4
collaborative learning approach, 229

Committee on Accreditation of
    Canadian Medical Schools
    (CACMS), 69
communication
  with consultants, 98–9
  with nurses, 97–8
communication skills, 65–6, 83–4,
    228
community settings, 193–4
computer as teaching tool, 72–84
conceptualization, 51
constructive criticism, *see*
    constructive feedback
constructive feedback, 45, 63, 188
constructivism, 4
consultants, communication with,
    98–9
content knowledge, 194
"conversational" question, 176
core content talk, 169–70
Council of Residency Directors
    for Emergency Medicine
    (CORD), 197, 203, 204
course directorships, 26
creative teaching activities, 150
criticism, 153
curriculum design, 4
customized program, developing,
    195–7

debriefing, 40, 111
decision-making responsibility,
    229–30
dedicated teaching shifts, 128–30
demonstrative style, 163
diagnostic imaging, 76–8
didactic curriculum, 143–4
didactic educational component,
    122–3
didactic lecture, 163
"difficult" ED Patient, 149, 150
distance education, 195
drugs toxicity, interactions, and
    treatment, 79–80

ECG analysis, 78–9
ED STAT! teaching model, 205, 214
educational activities
    implementation, 11–12
    planning, 11
educational feedback, *see* feedbacks,
        in ED
"educational nirvana", 138
educational objectives and
        curriculum, 109–10
educational prescription cards, 21
*Educational Researcher*, 202
educational Resources Information
        Center (ERIC), 201, 202
effective teachers, 194, 213–14, 221
    in chaotic environment, 136
    characteristics, 9
    qualities, 108
EMedHome.com, 195, 196
eMedicine, 195, 196
emergency medicine education, 30
Emergency Medicine Foundation
        (EMF), 203, 204
emergency physicians (EP), 30, 35,
        90, 98, 195, 228
    medical education websites of,
        196
emergency ultrasound, 30
EMF/ACEP Teaching Fellowship,
        204
encouragement of learners, 19–20
enthusiasm, 39, 108, 175, 184, 226
environment for learning
    interpersonal/relationship
        environment, 8–10
    physical environment, 8
environmental adjuncts, 164–5
environmental obstacles, 165
Essential Procedures in Emergency
        Medicine (EPEM), 57
evaluation of learners, 12–13
evaluation plan for patient, 111
evaluation versus feedback, 70
evidence-based medicine, 135

experience cycle versus explanation
        cycle, 39–41

face-to-face debriefing, 54
face-to-face meetings, 142
facial expression, 175
facilitator, 7, 11
    characteristics, 183–4
    feedback for, 190
    techniques
        brainstorming, 185–6
        preparation, 184–5
        questioning, 185
        restraint, 185
        summarization, 185
        tension level, adjusting, 186, 188
factual questioning, 228
faculty development, as guide, 22,
        192
    academic setting, practicing in,
        193–4
    assistant resources
        formal faculty development
            programs, 202–5
        online materials, 199–202
        printed materials, 198–9
        professional societies, 197–8
    clinicians as teachers, 194
    customized program, developing,
        195–7
    definition, 192–3
    goals setting, 194–5
    pifalls, 206
    promotion, 205–6
faculty–resident interaction, 137
"feedback sandwich", 63
feedbacks, 109–10, 153, 178, 222,
        231–2
    additional methods and tools
        accreditation process, 69
        faculty/trainee development,
            69–70
        feedback cards, 67
        feedback versus evaluation, 70

formal feedback sessions, 68–9
written feedback/evaluation,
    67–8
definition, 60
general guidelines, 61
    areas, focus on, 64–5
    constructive feedback,
        providing, 63
    incorporation into teaching
        models, 66–7
    joint venture, making, 66
    nonjudgmental and non-
        evaluative language, 65–6
    positive feedback, providing, 62
    self-assessment, eliciting, 63–4
    specific behaviors/actions,
        observations of, 62–3
    strategies for improvement,
        developing, 67
    timing, 64
    in learning process, 53–4
"finalizing" ED patient visit, 149–50
focused teaching point, 219–22
formal didactics, 118
formal faculty development
    programs, 202–5
formal feedback sessions, 68–9
fourth year (senior level) medical
    students (MS4s), 146
future generation physicians,
    training, 26–8

General Emergency Medicine, 196
Glasgow Coma Score, 82
goals setting
    for learners, 10–11
    in faculty development, 194–5
good teaching points, 220, 222
Google, 73, 199
Google Scholar, 75
great teachers, 159
    environmental adjuncts and
        barriers, 164–5
    learners' expectations, 160–61

medical educators, considerations
    of, 161–3
teaching styles, 163–4
ground rules setting, 176
guided practice, 51, 53–4

hand-on-hand contact, 53
Harvard Macy Institute, 205
Human Chorionic Gonadotropin
    (HCG) measurement, 83

independent learning, 21, 195, 229
individual resident experience,
    tailoring
    continuity of learning,
        improving, 142–3
    didactic curriculum, 143–4
    remediation, 143
informal didactic teaching
    approach, 117–18, 122
information filtration, 109
inspiration and information,
    importance of, 21–2
instructor preparation, 50
instructor-based obstacles, 18
instructor-to-student ratio, 51
interactive discussion, 20, 52
interactive style of teaching, 163
interpersonal environment, for
    learning, 8–10
interview-synthesis-investigation-
    management, 216

*Journal of General Internal Medicine*,
    199

knowledge retention, encouraging,
    139–40
Knowles, Malcolm, 5

laser pointer, 175–6
leadership, continuity of, 127–8
"learn by observation", 229
learner-based obstacles, 18–19

learner-centered activities, 162–3, 163–4
learner centered instruction, 38
learners
    activation, 228–9
    assessment, 153–4
    diagnosing, 218
    self-assessment, 63–4
learning
    as adult, 5–7
    as child, 4
    continuity of, 142–3
    process
        conceptualization, 51
        guided practice, 53–4
        verbalization, 52–3
        visualization, 51–2
    theories, 4
lecture-based curricula, 36, 118
Liaison Committee on Medical Education (LCME), 69
life threatening moments, 12
likelihood ratios, 76, 78
literature review session, 182
Luber, Sam, 199, 200

master educator, 26
    benefits of teaching, in EM
        future emergency physician, training, 26–8
        local, regional, and national organizations, forming backbone of, 29
        specific areas of interest, 28–9
medical decision making, 137, 219
Medical Education Research Certification program, 205
medical education websites, of emergency physicians, 196
medical search engines, 75
medical simulation, 28
medical students, teaching, 105–6
    clinical teaching, 110–12

educational objectives and curriculum, 109–10
effective teacher, qualities of, 108
overwhelming, prevention of student from, 112
philosophy, teaching, 108–9
problems, in EM, 107–8
uniqueness, in EM, 106–7
mentoring process, 27, 28
"micro teaching", 204
microskills model, of clinical teaching, 41, 163–4, 214–15
models, of teaching, 54–6, 119, 214–15
    for off-service residents, 115
        bedside teaching, 116–17
        formal didactics, 118
        informal didactic teaching approach, 117–18
    practical tips for improvement
        didactics educational component, 122–3
        effective bedside educator, 119–21
moderator's goal, 186
motivation, for teaching EM, 24–5
MS4s, see fourth year (senior level) medical students
multitasking teaching, 141

National Center for Emergency Medicine Infomatics (NCEMI), 77, 196
networking, 197
NIH stroke scale, 81
non-EM trainees, 115
non-English speaking patients, fluent translators for, 83–4
non-procedural clinical teaching, see resident physicians, education of
nonthreatening questions, 228
nonverbal behavior, 174–5
nurses, communication with, 97–8

Objective Structured Clinical
Examinations (OSCEs), 45
obstacles in teaching, 16
frequent interruptions, 17
instructor-based obstacles, 18
learner-based obstacles, 18–19
limited physical space for
teaching, 17
solutions
encouragement of learners,
21–2
faculty development programs,
investment in, 22
shared responsibility, 20
spontaneous teaching activities,
preparation for, 20–21
teaching techniques usage,
19–20
time limitations, 16–17
off-service curriculum, 116
off-service residents, teaching
models for, 115
bedside teaching, 116–17
formal didactics, 118
informal didactic teaching
approach, 117–18
off-service trainees, 115, 116, 118
educational objectives and goals
for, 119, 120
practical strategies for, 120–21
One Minute Clinical Preceptor, 66
"one-minute teaching" strategy,
165
one-on-one discussion, 186, 229
online calculators, 82
online educational modules, 122
online materials, 199–202
online resources, 72, 77
online scores, 82
open and respectful relationship,
8–10
open questions, 185
oral assessment, in group
discussion, 190

oral examination cases, 187
"oral wisdom" of educators, 198
organized communication, 173
orientation, 10, 110
Ottawa Ankle Rule, 222
over-teaching, 38, 39
OVID, 75

participation, assessing, 190
passive learning, 41
patient care and safety, improving,
29–30
patient encounter
initial encounter, 90, 92
initial interview, closing, 94
patient-centred interview, 92–4
visit, concluding, 94–7
patient–physician interaction, 231
patient preparation, in learning
environment, 50
patient-centred interview, 92–4
patients flow and acuity,
approaches to, 136–8
Patients/Interventions/
Comparisons/Outcomes
(PICO) model, 75
pattern recognition, 139
pearls and pitfalls, in teaching, 225
decision-making responsibility,
229–30
expectations clarification, 226–7
feedback, providing, 231–2
learners, activating, 228–9
needs of audiences, determining,
227
right reasons, 226
safe learning, practice of, 230–31
simplicity, making, 230
teaching methods, 227–8
thought process, conveying, 231
pedagogical learning, 5
pedagogy, 4
personal and professional growth,
88–9

personality traits, 65, 88
  of bedside teachers, 37
philosophy, of teaching, 108–9
physical contact, 92
physical environment, for learning,
  8
physicians, teaching, *see* resident
    physicians, education of
pimping, 41, 227, 228
pitfalls
  in academics, 206
  and pearls in teaching    225
    decision-making responsibility,
      229–30
    expectations clarification,
      226–7
    feedbacks, providing, 231–2
    learners, activating, 228–9
    needs of audiences,
      determining, 227
    right reasons, 226
    safe learning, practice of,
      230–31
    simplicity, making, 230
    teaching methods, 227–8
    thought process, conveying,
      231
  in resident teaching, 150–53
PORT score, 82
positive discussions, 90
positive feedback, 62
post-test probability, 78
practice-based learning and
    improvement, 135–6
practicing, before presentation,
    177–8
pregnancy, changes and radiation
    risks in, 82–3
preparation
  for small group discussion, 184–5
  for teaching and learning
    procedures, 48–51
presentation skills, 168
  audience, understanding, 171

beginning, of talk, 172
  body language, knowing, 174–5
  end of talk, 171
  environment, aware of, 175–6
  ground rules setting, 176
  material, knowing, 172–3
  practice, 177–8
  stage fright, dealing with, 177
  talks, types of, 169–70
  voice and tone, attention to,
    173–4
pre-test probability, 78
"primum no nocere", 141
printed materials, for learning,
    198–9
problem-based learning (PBL), 183
problem-centered learning, 5
procedures, in teaching
  learning process, 51–4
  preparation, to teach and learn,
    48–51
  procedural education, creating,
    57–8
  small group discussions, 182
  theory-based framework, 54–6
Professional and Organizational
    Network for Higher
    Education, 192, 200
professional behavior, 88, 108
professional societies, 197–8
professionalism, 135
professionalism and interpersonal
    skills/communication, 87
  communication
    with consultant, 98–9
    with nurses, 97–8
  continual growth, promoting
    openness to, 88–9
  feedback, providing, 89–90, 91
  good work, acknowledging, 99
  motivation, providing, 88
  patient encounter
    initial encounter, 90, 92
    initial interview, closing, 94

professionalism and interpersonal
skills/communication,
(*continued*)
    patient-centred interview, 92–4
    visit, concluding, 94–7
    role model, 99
    standards and expectations
        setting, 89
    students, difficulties of, 99–100
Program for Physician–Educators,
    205
promotion and tenure guidelines,
    205–6
PubMed, 75

questioning, 185

radiology, 196
reflection in learning, 7
rehearsal, before presentation, 178
relationship setting, 8–10
residency office, 125–7
residency program, culture and
    conflicts of, 130–31
Residency Review Committee–
    Emergency Medicine
    (RRC–EM), 135–6
Residency Review Committees
    (RRC), 114
residency teaching triangle, *see*
    "educational nirvana"
resident errors, 141–2
resident physicians, education of
    ACGME core competencies, 132
        practice-based learning and
            improvement, 135–6
        professionalism, 135
        system-based practice, 132,
            134–5
    clinical teaching paradigms, for
        EM faculty
        "educational nirvana", 138
        effective teachers, in chaotic
            environment, 136

knowledge retention,
    encouraging, 139–40
multitasking teaching, 141
patients flow and acuity,
    approaches to, 136–8
pattern recognition, 139
resident errors, 141–2
visual diagnosis, 139
individual resident experience,
    tailoring
    continuity of learning,
        improving, 142–3
    didactic curriculum, 143–4
    remediation, 143
residency infrastructure and
    support
    dedicated teaching shifts,
        128–30
    leadership, continuity of,
        127–8
    residency office, 125–7
    residency program culture and
        conflicts, 130–31
    scheduling and effects, 128
teaching, 125, 146
    challenges, 146, 147
    expectations setting, 146–50
    learner assessment, 153–4
    organizational tool, to monitor
        patient progress, 154
    pitfalls, 150–53
    "teaching skill set", 146, 147
respect, 7
role modeling, 13–14, 89, 90, 100,
    161, 223
role-playing technique, 182–3, 186

Sackett Sandwich, 42
safe learning, practice of, 230–31
scheduling, of residents and faculty,
    128
scholarly activity, 193
scripts, for teaching, 222
search engines, 75

search terms, in Google, 199
seasoned veteran, 26
SEGUE Framework checklist, 90, 92
self-assessment, 63–4
   *see also* self-directed learning
self-directed learning, 5, 6
shared responsibility, 20
shift card, 142
sign-out rounds, 229
simulation-based medical
   education, 29
simulator model, 55
skill acquisition, 53–4
skin lesions, systematic approach
   to, 80–81
small group discussion skills, 180
   assessment, 190
   benefits, 180–81
   case-based learning, 182
   challenges and solutions
      experience into lecture format,
         converting, 189
      participation, 189
      preventing one participant,
         from dominating, 189
   facilitators
      characteristics of, 183–4
      techniques of, 184–6
   goals establishment, 186
   group, sizing, 186
   literature review session, 182
   problem-based learning (PBL),
      183
   role-playing technique, 182–3
   rules and expectations, setting,
      188
   seating arrangement, 186–7
   selecting materials, 187
   skill set, developing, 181
   staying on task, 189–90
   teaching procedures, 182
Society for Academic Emergency
   Medicine (SAEM), 28, 196,
   198, 201, 204

speakers, characteristics of, 197
speaking, 179
   environment, aware of, 175–6
specific behaviors/actions,
   observations of, 62–3
spontaneous teaching activities,
   preparation for, 20–21
stage fright, 177
standard of care, defining, 29–30
Standardized Direct Observation
   Assessment Tool, 45
Stanford University, 205
STAT teaching model, 205, 214,
   218–19
structured risk assessment, 82
student
   evaluation, 12–13, 57–8
   professionalism and
      communication, difficulty
      with, 99–100
   promoting reflection in, 110
   style of teaching, 163–4
summarization, in small group
   discussions, 185
system-based practice, 132

talks, types of, 169–70
task analysis, 50
"teach-only" attending approach, 39
teachable moments, 111
teacher–learner discussions, 117
teacher–student interaction, 227
teacher-centered impediments,
   164–5
teachers, *see* bedside teachers;
   effective teachers; great
   teachers
"teaching attending", 121, 122, 129
"teaching bite", 38, 39
teaching, in EM
   beginning educator, 25
   benefits
      future emergency physician,
         training, 26–8

teaching, in EM (*continued*)
  local organizations, backbone
    formation of, 29
  national organizations,
    backbone formation of, 29
  regional organizations,
    backbone formation of, 29
  specific areas of interest, 28–9
  future, foundations for, 30
  master educator, 26
  motivation, 24–5
  patient care and safety, improving
    standard of care, defining,
    29–30
  seasoned veteran, 26
teaching methods, 227–8
teaching models, *see* models, of
  teaching
teaching scripts, 222
"teaching skill set", 146, 147
teaching styles, in ED setting, 163–4
teaching techniques, to overcome
  obstacles in ED, 19–20
tension level, adjusting, 186, 188
The Academic Assembly, 204
theory-based framework, 54–6
thought process, conveying, 231
"time triage", 8
time-honored technique, 140
timing, 159
  of feedback, 64
toxicology, 80

trainees, teaching, 114
  non-EM trainees, 115
  off-service residents, teaching
    models for, 115
    bedside teaching, 116–17
    formal didactics, 118
    informal didactic teaching
      approach, 117–18
  teaching models, practical tips
    to, 119
  didactics educational
    component, enhancing,
    122–3
  effective bedside educator,
    119–21

"unconditional positive regard", 89
uninterrupted teaching rounds, 39
university settings, 193

verbal discussion, *see* evaluation of
  learners
verbalization, 51, 52–3
visual diagnosis, 139
visualization, 51–2

Wagner, Mary Jo, 199, 200
websites, recommended, 84
Well's criteria, 82
work rounds, 137
working knowledge phase, 40
written feedback/evaluation, 67–8